"The concept of glycemic index is key to under[...] drate on human health. *The New Glucose Revolution*, written by leading scientists, conveys this information clearly, thoroughly, and convincingly."
—**WALTER WILLETT, MD, PhD,** Professor of Epidemiology and Nutrition, Harvard School of Public Health, on *The New Glucose Revolution*

"This is the best diet book. . . . I recommend it above all others."—**JEAN CARPER,** best-selling author of *Miracle Cures* and *USA Weekend* columnist, on *The Low GI Diet Revolution*

"Written by leading authorities in nutrition . . . this program is simple, practical, and powerful. I recommend it with enthusiasm."—**DAVID S. LUDWIG, MD, PhD,** Director, Obesity Program & Optimal Weight for Life (OWL) clinic, Children's Hospital Boston, on *The Low GI Diet Revolution*

"Written by the world's experts on diet and the glycemic index, this book will provide the tools you need to make dietary and lifestyle changes to achieve lifelong health."—**JOANN E. MANSON, MD, DrPH,** Professor of Medicine, Harvard Medical School, Chief of Division of Preventive Medicine, Brigham and Women's Hospital, on *The New Glucose Revolution for Diabetes*

"The concept of the glycemic index has been distorted and bastardized by popular writers and diet gurus. Here, at last, is a book that explains what we know about the glycemic index and its importance in designing a diet for optimum health."—**ANDREW WEIL, MD,** University of Arizona College of Medicine, author of *Eating Well for Optimum Health*, on *The New Glucose Revolution*

"This book clearly explains that there are different kinds of carbohydrates that work in different ways and why a universal recommendation to 'increase the carbohydrate content of your diet' is plainly simple and scientifically accurate. Everyone should put the glycemic index approach into practice."
—**ARTEMIS P. SIMOPOULOS, MD,** senior author of *The Omega Diet* and *The Healing Diet* and President, Center for Genetics, Nutrition and Health, Washington, DC, on *The New Glucose Revolution*

"*The Glucose Revolution* is nutrition science for the 21st century. Clearly written, it gives the scientific rationale for why all carbohydrates are not created equal. It is a practical guide for both professionals and patients. The food suggestions and recipes are exciting and tasty."—**RICHARD N. PODELL, MD, MPH,** Clinical Professor, Department of Family Medicine, UMDNJ-Robert Wood Johnson Medical School, and coauthor of *The G-Index Diet: The Missing Link That Makes Permanent Weight Loss Possible*, on *The Glucose Revolution*

**THE EXPERIMENT**

BECAUSE EVERY BOOK IS A TEST OF NEW IDEAS

# The
# LOW GI
## Eating Plan for an
## Optimal Pregnancy

*The Authoritative Science-Based Nutrition*
*Guide for Mother and Baby*

DR. JENNIE BRAND-MILLER,
DR. KATE MARSH AND DR. ROBERT MOSES

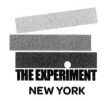

THE EXPERIMENT
NEW YORK

THE LOW GI EATING PLAN FOR AN OPTIMAL PREGNANCY: *The Authoritative Science-Based Nutrition Guide for Mother and Baby*

First published in Australia in 2012 as *The Bump to Baby Diet: Low GI Eating Plan for Conception, Pregnancy and Beyond* by Hachette Australia Pty Ltd. This North American edition is published by arrangement with Hachette Australia Pty Ltd.

The Experiment, LLC
260 Fifth Avenue, Suite 3 South
New York, NY 10001-6408
theexperimentpublishing.com

The Experiment's books are available at special discounts when purchased in bulk for premiums and sales promotions as well as for fundraising or educational use. For details, contact us at info@theexperimentpublishing.com.

Library of Congress Cataloging-in-Publication Data

[Bump to baby diet]
    The low GI eating plan for an optimal pregnancy : the authoritative science-based nutrition guide for mother and baby / Dr. Jennie Brand-Miller, Dr. Kate Marsh, Dr. Robert Moses.
        pages cm
    Revision of: Bump to baby diet. 2012.
    Includes bibliographical references and index.
    ISBN 978-1-61519-082-9 (pbk.) -- ISBN 978-1-61519-174-1 (ebook) 1. Pregnancy--Nutritional aspects. 2. Mothers--Nutrition. 3. Glycemic index. I. Marsh, Kate. II. Moses, Robert, 1946- III. Title.
    RG559.B715 2013
    618.2'42--dc23
                              2012042033

ISBN 978-1-61519-082-9
Ebook ISBN 978-1-61519-174-1

Cover design by Howard Grossman
Cover photograph © iStockphoto I Kupicoo Images
Text design by Liz Seymour, Seymour Designs
Typesetting by Neuwirth & Associates, Inc.
Manufactured in the United States of America
Distributed by Workman Publishing Company, Inc.
Distributed simultaneously in Canada by Thomas Allen & Son Ltd.

First published April 2013
10 9 8 7 6 5 4 3 2 1

*This book is dedicated to our patients and study volunteers, whose questions and welfare have fostered further research, and to all women, who, by reading this book, may improve their pregnancy experience and future quality of life*

Jennie, Kate and Bob

# Contents

# PART 5 Recipes

# Introduction

## A PREGNANCY BOOK LIKE NO OTHER

This book about eating for a healthy pregnancy is at the cutting edge of science and medicine. Most pregnancy books will cover nutrition requirements, supplements, foods to emphasize and foods to avoid. This book does that too, but it goes much further. *The Low GI Eating Plan for an Optimal Pregnancy* has a unique focus on the importance of your weight at the start of pregnancy, your weight gain over the next nine months and your baby's birth weight, and the profound effect these have on the future health of you and your baby. The GI, a way of rating the carbs in your diet, is for everybody, but it's especially relevant during pregnancy, and this book is aimed squarely at women who are pregnant—or planning to be.

*The Low GI Eating Plan for an Optimal Pregnancy* is not a fad diet, but a safe and healthy action plan for eating before and during pregnancy with many proven "value-added" benefits. A low GI diet is one in which

### What is the GI?

GI stands for "glycemic index." It's a scale from 0 to 100 that helps guide carbohydrate choices and is a physiologically based measure of the effect of carbohydrates on blood glucose levels. It provides an easy and delicious way to eat a healthy diet and at the same time control fluctuations in blood glucose. After testing hundreds of foods around the world, scientists have now found that foods with a low GI will have less of an effect on blood glucose levels than foods with a high GI.

meals have a lower blood glucose impact. In addition to optimizing your weight gain and nutrient intake throughout pregnancy, you control your blood glucose levels and reduce the chances of developing gestational diabetes or having a complicated delivery.

Pregnancy is a stage in life when the carbohydrates in food play a starring role. This is because your average blood glucose level throughout the day is directly correlated with your baby's growth rate in the womb. Quite simply, glucose is the primary fuel that drives all aspects of your baby's development. If your glucose levels are too high then your baby will grow too fast and be born with excessive amounts of body fat. This is not a new finding. It's the main reason why women who have type 1 diabetes (a condition that requires daily insulin injections to maintain normal glucose levels) are given close medical attention before and during their pregnancies. It's also the principal reason why all pregnant women are routinely screened during pregnancy to determine if they have developed gestational diabetes. What's new is that we now know that even mildly elevated glucose levels during pregnancy can have serious consequences.

Even mildly elevated glucose levels during pregnancy can have serious consequences.

Pregnancy is a like a metabolic stress test. Even during the first trimester, your placenta and growing baby draw so much glucose from your bloodstream that your early morning glucose levels are lower than they are in the nonpregnant state. Pregnant women use carbohydrates at a greater rate both at rest and during exercise than do nonpregnant women, so one of the first metabolic adaptations your body makes to pregnancy is a greater capacity to produce glucose in the liver. While this makes perfect sense (if your access to food is temporarily restricted, your growing baby will still be getting the energy it needs), it means that glucose synthesis is always "on" and thus all women become more resistant to insulin's effects as pregnancy progresses. For some women, this precipitates gestational diabetes.

Pregnancy is also a time when women often gain too much weight, compromising not only their own future health, but that of their baby. Traditionally, dietary advice for pregnancy has focused on making sure there's adequate intake of all the essential nutrients. That's not surprising considering the fact that the requirements for many nutrients are higher than at any other time in life. Unfortunately, weight gain during pregnancy, despite its importance, is not given the emphasis that it deserves. In this book, we show you how to calculate your ideal weight gain (depending on your height and pre-pregnancy weight) and how to monitor it and keep it under your control.

One of the reasons we wrote this book is because infant birth weights and child obesity have increased hand in hand over recent decades in most industrialized nations. We now know that life inside the womb is a critical period for the metabolic "programming" of obesity in later life. Your weight at the time of conception and weight gain from early to late pregnancy profoundly influence your infant's birth weight and future risk of becoming overweight. Reducing the GI of your diet is one of the safest and most effective ways of ensuring that your baby grows at the optimum rate without laying down excessive body fat.

*The Low GI Eating Plan for an Optimal Pregnancy* is the only low GI diet book specifically for pregnancy written by internationally recognized scientists qualified in nutrition, dietetics and diabetes, and at the cutting edge of research on carbohydrates, the GI and pregnancy. We understand the connection between food, maternal blood glucose levels and your baby's future health. Our training and experience give us the tools to help pregnant women beat excessive weight gain, without compromising nutrition, during this important stage of life.

The figures speak for themselves. The New Glucose Revolution series is a bestseller around the world, with 3.5 million copies in print in more than twelve languages. We publish in the world's leading nutrition and medical journals first, then we show you how to put it into practice. You can be reassured that our dietary advice is a safe, balanced and sustainable way of eating that puts no one at risk in either the short or long term.

*The Low GI Eating Plan for an Optimal Pregnancy* is based on choosing carbohydrates that are slowly digested and absorbed, producing only gentle rises and falls in blood sugar (blood glucose) and insulin levels. It is not a low-carb diet, not a low-fat diet, not even a high-protein diet. It's much more flexible and sustainable than any of those, and it is quite simply a delicious way of eating. We promise you won't be ravenously hungry between meals, you won't be weighing out food and you certainly won't be counting calories. One of the reasons this diet is easy is its unique ability to keep you feeling fuller for longer. It helps control appetite by controlling blood glucose and stimulating the production of the body's own natural appetite suppressants. Metabolically, it reduces insulin levels and maximizes the burning of fat. It's not restrictive or monotonous, and it includes your favorite foods, or foods that could easily become your favorites.

A low GI diet is a delicious way of eating... You won't be ravenously hungry between meals, you won't be weighing out food and you certainly won't be counting calories.

In a nutshell, by following the Low GI Eating Plan, you can eat and enjoy moderate amounts of lean meat, poultry, fish, shellfish, eggs, and low-fat dairy or soy foods such as milk, tofu, soy milk, cheese and yogurt, and reasonable quantities of bread, pasta, breakfast cereal, rice noodles and grains (such as quinoa and barley). Legumes play a starring role because they have the lowest GI of all and are particularly important if you are vegetarian. You can also eat large portions of non-starchy vegetables and salads, and moderate amounts of fruit and starchy vegetables. Your salads, will be dressed with vinaigrettes made with healthy oils. You'll have three balanced meals a day, and we encourage you to have morning and afternoon snacks. You can even include the occasional dessert or other indulgence.

This is a special book for another important reason—it deals not just with energy intake (what you eat) but energy output—energy expenditure and physical activity. This is the critical side of the energy equation, the part that many pregnancy books ignore. Unless you increase your level of activity, weight gain during pregnancy will inevitably exceed the recommendation. Exercising is not only healthy for you and your baby, but by exercising more, you can reap the benefits of more muscle tone and joie de vivre, making it easier to regain your pre-pregnancy figure, and reduce your odds of developing gestational diabetes and having a difficult delivery.

If you're finding it hard to become pregnant, this diet will help to increase your chances by getting right to the root of one of the problems—insulin resistance—that affects about one in five women. We take you by the hand, describing exactly what you need to do and eat to maximize your fertility as well as your baby's future health. You'll learn the skills necessary to achieving a serious, sustainable lifestyle change—the key to lifelong health. We show you how to embrace simple forms of physical activity and behavioral control that will keep the engine revving and stop unwanted weight gain. You'll be taking care of yourself, looking good, feeling good and maximizing your own health as well as your baby's. Physical activity and healthy food habits will become just that—*habits* that are easy to sustain.

This is a family-friendly diet, too: Your partner and your other children will be sitting down to the same delicious food as you; the quantities alone will vary. Unlike many fad diets, there are no issues with long-term threats to bones, kidneys, blood vessels and heart health.

All this good advice comes to you from the world's most recognized experts on the GI of foods.

## WHO ARE WE?

JENNIE BRAND-MILLER is Professor of Human Nutrition at the University of Sydney in Sydney, Australia. She holds a Personal Chair in the School of Molecular Bioscience and leads the nutrition division of the Boden Institute of Obesity, Nutrition, Exercise & Eating Disorders. Affectionately known as "the queen of the glycemic index," she is acknowledged worldwide for her expertise on carbohydrates and health. Her research interests focus on many areas of nutrition, diet and diabetes, insulin resistance, lactose intolerance and infant nutrition. She holds a special interest in evolutionary nutrition and the diet of hunter-gatherers. It was her early research on Australian Aboriginal bush foods that inspired her to start looking at differences between modern and traditional diets as a cause of the "diseases of affluence" such as diabetes. In 1981, the very first paper to mention the glycemic index accidentally landed on her desk, precipitating a project for an honors student. Since then, Jennie and her team have played a key role on the world stage in establishing the scientific validity, benefits and practicalities of the glycemic index. Twenty books and more than 220 peer-reviewed journal articles over a space of thirty years make her eminently qualified to give you all the facts you need to put a healthy low GI diet into practice.

**DR. KATE MARSH** is an Advanced Accredited Practicing Dietitian and Credentialed Diabetes Educator with a Masters of Nutrition and Dietetics from the University of Sydney and a Graduate Certificate in Diabetes Education and Management from the University of Technology, Sydney. She has recently completed her PhD at the University of Sydney, looking at the benefits of a low GI diet in the management of insulin resistance in women with polycystic ovary syndrome (PCOS), and has published a number of scientific papers. Kate works in private practice in Sydney, Australia, and has a particular interest in PCOS and diabetes, including gestational diabetes, having worked with thousands of women with these conditions over the years.

She chairs a PCOS discussion group for dietitians, cochairs a diabetes interest group for dietitians and has been involved in the development of evidence-based practice guidelines for the management of PCOS and type 1 diabetes in Australia. Kate is also coauthor of *The Low GI Guide to Living Well with PCOS, The New Glucose Revolution Low GI Vegetarian Cookbook* and *The New Glucose Revolution Low GI Gluten-Free Eating Made Easy*, and writes regularly for a number of magazines on diabetes, PCOS, insulin resistance and vegetarian nutrition.

**PROFESSOR ROBERT MOSES** is Clinical Professor at the University of Wollongong, and Director of Diabetes Services for the Illawarra Shoalhaven Local Health District. He has more than thirty-five years of experience with the clinical problems of people with diabetes and is an acknowledged national and international authority on the topic of diabetes and pregnancy. He has researched and published extensively on the problems of gestational diabetes and has always had a great interest and enthusiasm for the beneficial effects of a low GI diet during pregnancy. Robert has also been on the editorial board and is an associate editor of the world's leading clinical diabetes scientific journal. In this capacity he has early access to a major portion of the best research and discussion about the problems of diabetes in pregnancy.

## HOW TO USE THIS BOOK

This book is divided into five sections. If you are still in the planning stages ("just practicing"), then Part 1 is written especially for you. If you're already pregnant, then skip straight to Part 2 for all the information on what to eat, weight gain, blood glucose, diabetes in pregnancy and exercise. Part 3 deals with all things relevant to postdelivery, but it would be useful to read it now so you're prepared once baby is born. Part 4 covers the practical side of what to eat (putting it all on the plate) and has more than fifty delicious recipes to give you a head start. At the back of the book you'll find a weight-gain chart, which you can photocopy or tear out and put on your fridge. Finally, because we are scientists as well as authors, we list all our resources and references should you need further information. We wish you healthy eating and happy reading!

JENNIE, KATE AND BOB

# Glossary

### DIABETES–GESTATIONAL
Gestational diabetes refers to any degree of "glucose intolerance" diagnosed for the first time during pregnancy.

### DIABETES–TYPE 1
An autoimmune disease where the pancreas does not produce any insulin and sufferers are reliant upon insulin injections to maintain a balanced blood glucose level.

### DIABETES–TYPE 2
A disease that develops when the body begins having problems producing insulin. For a long time the body will struggle to make extra insulin to overcome the problem, but eventually people with type 2 diabetes develop a shortage of insulin. People with type 2 diabetes need to make the best use of the insulin they have and make it last as long as possible. Tablets or insulin injections may be necessary.

### GI
The abbreviation for the glycemic index, a measure of the effect of carbohydrates on blood glucose levels.

### GLUCOSE TOLERANCE TEST (GTT)
A test used to diagnose diabetes at any time during pregnancy. The test, often given at the start of the third trimester, requires an overnight fast (nothing to eat), followed by a blood test, a drink of a glucose solution and then blood tests after one and two hours.

### INSULIN RESISTANCE
An insensitivity of the body to the action of insulin, a hormone which is important in regulating blood glucose levels.

## LISTERIOSIS

A serious infection caused by the *Listeria* bacteria, which is found naturally in some foods. If the infection passes on to your unborn baby, it can cause miscarriage or stillbirth.

## NEURAL TUBE DEFECT (NTD)

An opening in the spinal cord or brain that should have closed during development, which can lead to a condition known as spina bifida.

## POLYCYSTIC OVARY SYNDROME (PCOS)

Polycystic ovary syndrome is a hormonal disorder affecting between 5 and 10 percent of women before menopause, which is linked with insulin resistance and type 2 diabetes and can affect fertility and increase the risk of developing gestational diabetes.

## POSTPARTUM

Following childbirth.

## POSTPARTUM DEPRESSION (PPD)

Depression that occurs within the first year after having a baby.

## SALMONELLOSIS

Illness caused by the food poisoning bacterial *Salmonella*, which can cause miscarriage. While many foods can be infected, high-risk foods include raw or undercooked eggs (which may be incorporated into commercial and homemade sauces and desserts), chicken and other poultry and bean sprouts.

## TOXOPLASMOSIS

Disease caused by the parasite *Toxoplasma gondii*, which can harm your unborn child. The most common cause of infection for humans is close contact with an infected cat, but raw meat and unpasteurized goat's milk are also a risk.

# PART 1
# Planning your pregnancy

*We all want our children to be born healthy, but few of us understand the extent to which we can influence our child's future health even before they are conceived. If you are thinking about starting a family or if you've been trying hard to conceive, but are not there yet, then this section is for you.*

*Here we explain exactly why it makes good sense to optimize your health before conceiving. We outline the ins and outs of a fertility-friendly diet, explaining the low GI lifestyle habits that will pay big dividends. We also answer frequently asked questions about supplements—whether you really need them, which ones are best and which should be avoided.*

# Chapter 1

# Optimizing your health and lifestyle

One of the major reasons we sat down to write this book is because one study after another is showing that a child's risk of obesity, type 2 diabetes and even heart disease can be influenced by their mother's lifestyle habits before conception. Hard to believe, we know, but it's undeniable and based on high-quality studies in both humans and animals. And while the focus tends to be on females, men aren't off the hook. Ideally, they, too, should be leading a healthy lifestyle at the time of conception.

## IT STARTS WITH IMPROVING YOUR OWN HEALTH

Adopting a healthy lifestyle, including a balanced low GI diet, before conceiving can improve fertility (that is, the ability to produce a healthy baby) in both men and women, as well as positively influencing a child's health before and after birth. Since most women don't know they are pregnant in the first vital weeks, being in good shape ensures you are providing your baby with the best possible environment in which to develop, right from day one. Here are the habits worth focusing on before you start trying to conceive.

## AIM FOR A HEALTHY WEIGHT

Ideally, women should be within a healthy weight range at the start of pregnancy. Of growing concern, however, is the fact that two thirds of women of reproductive age are overweight in the United States. In fact, excess weight in either partner reduces the chances of getting pregnant.

The children of overweight mothers are also more likely to be overweight themselves simply because of the conditions inside the womb. There are other health risks, too. Babies born to mothers who are carrying excess weight during pregnancy have higher levels of body fat and insulin resistance (the root of the problem in type 2 diabetes), even as newborns. Thus overweight mothers increase the risk of their child developing metabolic problems such as obesity, prediabetes and high cholesterol in their teenage years.

That's the bad news; now for the good news. You don't need to reach your ideal weight before you conceive: Research shows that losing as little as 5 or 6 pounds in the month or so before conception improves the chances of success and reduces health risks for you and your baby. You need to lose this weight wisely so that your overall nutrition is stable when it really matters: the moment of conception. Adopting healthy low GI eating habits, moderating your portion sizes and regular exercise will all do the trick. Avoid overly restrictive diets and rapid weight loss—instead, aim for a healthy, sustainable rate of weight loss of around 1 pound per week.

## OPTIMIZE YOUR EATING HABITS

Good nutrition is more about food quality than food quantity. Eating well prior to conception can improve the chances of conception and ensure that your nutritional stores are at optimum levels during those first vital minutes, days and weeks when your baby's organs are being formed. Sperm quality is also important. Researchers at Australia's University of New South Wales (UNSW) made world headlines with their groundbreaking research on the important role played by the father's diet. Their findings suggest that males who eat a poor diet, high in saturated fat, prior to conception will have daughters who show early signs of diabetes by the time of puberty. We now know that diet and other environmental factors have the ability to leave "marks" on the DNA (called epigenetic marks) that influence the regulation and transcription of those genes.

The father-to-be's diet also plays an important role.

## AVOID OR LIMIT ALCOHOL

No amount of alcohol is known to be safe during pregnancy. Since you won't know you are pregnant in the first few weeks, when your baby's organs are already starting to form, it is best to avoid alcohol when you are trying to conceive. Excessive alcohol intake affects both male and female fertility. We recommend that you stay on the safe side by avoiding alcohol while you are trying to conceive, but if you choose to drink, limit your intake to no more than two drinks in one day and no more than seven drinks in a week. Binge drinking poses the highest risk and should be avoided (whatever your plans!).

## IF YOU SMOKE, QUIT

We know this is very blunt (it's meant to be!). Smoking can reduce fertility in both males and females. Pregnant women who smoke have a higher risk of miscarriage, ectopic pregnancy (when the fertilized egg grows in the fallopian tube rather than in the uterus), premature birth and stillbirth. Babies born to smoking mothers also have a greater risk of sudden infant death syndrome (SIDS). Even exposure to secondhand smoke from your partner or others can increase the risk of SIDS and having a small (low-birth-weight) baby. And children of nonsmoking women whose partners smoked prior to conception have been found to have a higher risk of childhood cancer. These facts are the basis of state laws that prohibit smoking in many public places. Ideally, both partners should resolve to stop smoking well before the decision to start a family.

### Three ways to quit

Quitting smoking isn't easy and you'll need all the support you can get. Fortunately, there is plenty of support available. You could start by:

1. Visiting your primary care physician (PCP)
2. Calling (800) QUIT-NOW, where you can talk with a trained quit coach about quitting at no cost, twenty-four hours a day, seven days a week
3. Visiting cdc.gov/tobacco or smokefree.gov to access an array of self-help materials and find a smoking cessation support group near you.

## STOP RECREATIONAL DRUGS

If you use recreational drugs such as marijuana, heroin and amphetamine-type stimulants while you're pregnant, they will pass through your placenta to your baby. They may harm your baby directly or cause it to have withdrawal symptoms after birth. There is no safe level of drug use, for you or your unborn baby.

If you have a problem with any drug, whether prescribed or recreational, seek help as soon as possible. Visit samhsa.gov/treatment to search for the support options available to you, or see your PCP.

## REDUCE YOUR EXPOSURE TO HAZARDOUS CHEMICALS

While more research is needed, there is increasing evidence that exposure to hazardous substances during pregnancy may affect a child's long-term health. For this reason, it is best to avoid contact with chemicals such as lead-based paints (for example, avoid renovating an old house), herbicides, pesticides, solvents, aerosols and many household cleaning products, including oven cleaners and bleach, once you are trying to conceive. There are now many natural cleaning products available for all types of cleaning jobs, or good old baking soda and vinegar can do the job in many cases.

## GET MOVING

Exercise has many health benefits, regardless of your pregnancy plans, but if you are trying to conceive, improving your fitness improves your insulin sensitivity and helps your body cope better with the demands of pregnancy. In particular, exercising regularly before you get pregnant reduces your risk of developing gestational diabetes, a condition that requires careful medical supervision (see Chapter 7). Inactive women are much more likely to develop gestational diabetes. Considering the risks associated with gestational diabetes—including high birth weight babies, emergency Caesarean section and even stillbirth—you have every good reason to get moving!

Another reason to start some form of enjoyable physical activity before you conceive is that it will be easier to stick to an established routine once you're pregnant. Of course, depending on the type of exercise you are doing, you may need to make some modifications once pregnant—high impact activities (such as running, jumping or skipping) are associated with miscarriage in early pregnancy. Switching to lower impact exercise, such as swimming or walking, is a good choice. Exercises that carry any risk of injury (such as horseback riding or contact sports) are not recommended, and you may need to modify the intensity of exercise as your pregnancy progresses. In Chapter 8, we give you more details about appropriate type, amount and frequency of exercise during pregnancy.

Improving your fitness improves your insulin sensitivity and helps your body cope better with the demands of pregnancy.

### CUT DOWN ON CAFFEINE

A moderate intake of caffeine (two to three 8-ounce cups of coffee and three to five 8-ounce servings of tea or 12-ounce servings of caffeinated soft drinks) should not affect fertility, but too much caffeine during pregnancy may increase your chances of having a miscarriage, premature birth or a low-birth-weight baby. If you are a big consumer of caffeine, start cutting down gradually as soon as you begin trying to conceive. Remember that coffee, tea and soda aren't the only sources of caffeine— it is also found in energy drinks and chocolate. On page 52, you'll find the caffeine content of the most common drinks.

**YOUR PRE-CONCEPTION CHECK-UP**

Before you start trying to conceive, visit your doctor and discuss what you need to do to prepare. This will help to ensure you start your pregnancy in the best possible health. During this checkup, your doctor will want to address:

» Your lifestyle habits, including nutrition, exercise, alcohol, smoking and drug use—all the factors discussed above.

» Any current health problems you have that may need to be addressed before you try to conceive—for example, if you have diabetes (or a family history of diabetes), making sure your blood glucose levels are well controlled before you get pregnant is essential for reducing any risks to your baby.

» Reviewing any medications you are taking, including non-prescription medications and nutritional supplements. Some prescription medications haven't been tested for safety in pregnancy and may need to be ceased or changed. For example, many medications to treat high cholesterol, high blood pressure and diabetes cannot be taken in pregnancy. There are also many vitamin, mineral and herbal supplements that are not safe to take when you are pregnant, so don't take any supplements you're not sure about. You'll find more details on pages 32–33.

» Making sure your immunizations are up-to-date. If you become infected with German measles (rubella) while you're pregnant, it can harm your unborn baby. Even if you were vaccinated when younger, your immunity may be low by the time you are planning to start a family—a simple blood test can tell your doctor if your immunity is low. In this case you may need a rubella booster at least two to three months before you plan to become pregnant. Vaccinations for chickenpox (if you haven't previously been infected), whooping cough and influenza may also be recommended.

» Checking for any sexually transmitted disease (STDs). Not all STDs have obvious symptoms and some, like chlamydia, gonorrhea, or herpes, can make it harder to get pregnant or harm your unborn baby. If you have had an STD in the past, or you think you might be at risk of having an STD, tell your doctor so that you can decide together whether to be tested. STDs can be treated before you get pregnant.

» Discussing any diseases or disabilities that you or your partner have or that run in your family, and any abnormalities that your previous children have been born with.
» Having a dental checkup before you get pregnant is also a good idea, so you can avoid the need for treatments during pregnancy.

## ALREADY PREGNANT, BY CHANCE?

While planning your pregnancy has obvious benefits for you and your baby, we all know that things don't always go according to plan. So if you find yourself pregnant without any prior preparation, remember that nearly half of pregnancies in the United States are unplanned, and that the vast majority of babies are born healthy. From here on out, a healthy low GI lifestyle will still go a long way toward ensuring the best possible health for both you and your baby.

## STRUGGLING TO CONCEIVE—THE PCOS STORY

Polycystic ovary syndrome (PCOS) is an endocrine (hormonal) disorder affecting between 5 and 10 percent of women before menopause. Symptoms vary from one woman to the next but may include:

» Irregular or absent menstrual periods
» Infertility or reduced fertility
» Hirsutism (excess hair growth on the face, chest and stomach)
» Alopecia (scalp hair loss)
» Acne
» Obesity and difficulty losing weight
» Acanthosis nigricans (dark skin pigmentation around the neck and in the armpits)
» An increased risk of miscarriage.

One of the most common symptoms of PCOS is irregular or absent menstrual periods. For any one cycle, the lack of ovulation means an egg has not been released and conception can't take place. Hence, many women discover they have PCOS when they have trouble getting pregnant.

We now know that women with PCOS are also more likely to carry excess weight, particularly around the middle, one of the consequences of insulin resistance. Unfortunately, this extra weight can make the symptoms of PCOS worse and make it harder to become pregnant.

## THE INSULIN RESISTANCE LINK

Insulin resistance is an insensitivity of the body to the action of insulin. Insulin is a master hormone, secreted into the blood by the beta cells in the pancreas. One of insulin's most important functions is to regulate blood glucose levels. In many women with PCOS, the actions of insulin are blunted, so the body produces extra insulin to keep the blood glucose levels under control. High levels of insulin act on the ovaries to cause increased production of male hormones, which disrupts the normal ovulation cycle and causes many of the symptoms of PCOS (such as irregular or absent periods, acne and facial hair). High insulin levels also tend to promote fat storage, particularly around the middle, and can make weight loss more difficult. And because insulin resistance is the same underlying problem that occurs in type 2 diabetes, if you have PCOS, you are at greater risk of developing diabetes later in life, and are more likely to develop gestational diabetes when you are pregnant (we discuss this further in Chapter 7).

## LIFESTYLE CHANGES ARE KEY

Fortunately, it is not all bad news—in fact, diet, exercise and weight reduction all help to restore ovulation and improve fertility in women with PCOS, even with weight losses of as little as 5 to 6 pounds. It is for this reason that lifestyle changes are recommended as the first line of treatment for managing PCOS, before any medications are used.

While more research is needed to determine the best type of eating plan for PCOS, our own research has shown that a healthy low GI diet can go a long way toward improving insulin sensitivity and symptoms in women with PCOS.

If you have PCOS, making lifestyle changes before you try to conceive is particularly important. This will not only increase your chances of getting pregnant but will also reduce the risk of developing gestational diabetes when you do become pregnant and will set you on the path to prevent diabetes later in life.

# Chapter 2

# Fertility food—what you should (and shouldn't) be eating while trying to conceive

Your pre-conception eating plan should be aimed at maximizing your nutrient intake to ensure you start your pregnancy with a good store of important nutrients to support your pregnancy and for your baby to draw on. If you are overweight, aim for gradual weight loss on a balanced low GI diet. Avoid restrictive diets, particularly those that focus on a very high protein intake, include very little fat, or limit important food groups, such as fruit and vegetables.

Basically, you should be aiming for a healthy balanced diet containing a variety of foods from each of the major food groups and containing all of the essential nutrients your body needs to be in good shape to support a pregnancy. Of course, there are a few nutrients that warrant particular attention and also some foods you might consider limiting to optimize your fertility and to ensure your baby has the best possible environment to grow in from day one.

## A BALANCED LOW GI DIET

Forget fad diets when you are trying to conceive—restrictive diets of any kind may affect fertility and can also increase the likelihood that you start your pregnancy without adequate stores of important vitamins and minerals that you and your baby will need.

Instead of following a fad diet, aim to include a variety of foods from each of the main food groups each day. These include:

» Fruits and vegetables—aim for a variety of different types and colors
» Breads and cereals—choose whole grain varieties most of the time
» Protein foods including lean meat, poultry, fish, eggs, legumes, tofu, nuts and seeds
» Calcium-rich foods including milk, yogurt, cheese and calcium-fortified alternatives (such as fortified soy milk)
» Healthy fats including olive oil, avocado, nuts, seeds and nut/seed spreads.

## THE TOP FOUR NUTRIENTS FOR CONCEPTION

Having adequate levels of these four nutrients at the time of conception will ensure you start your pregnancy under the best possible circumstances. As we explain, some of these nutrients are particularly critical for your baby's early development at a time when you may not even know you are pregnant. If you make sure you are getting the right amount of each before you conceive, then you can guarantee your baby will also be getting enough from day one. The exact quantities needed before and during pregnancy, along with the best sources, are shown on page 206.

### FOLATE

Folate, or folic acid, is a B-group vitamin needed for normal growth and development but particularly for the development of the baby's brain, spinal cord and skeleton. Consuming enough folate in early pregnancy has been shown to reduce the risk of your baby developing birth defects such as neural tube defects (NTDs). We explain this further in Chapter 6. It is important to ensure you are getting enough at any given time, because you usually won't know you are pregnant in the first few weeks, when this nutrient matters most. It is recommended that you take folate for at least one month prior to conception. Foods rich in folate include green leafy vegetables such as spinach, broccoli, cabbage and brussels sprouts; legumes including lentils, chickpeas and dried beans; asparagus; avocado; nuts; oranges; wheat germ; and folate-fortified breads and cereals. Because even the most balanced modern diet may not provide sufficient folic acid for early pregnancy, folic acid supplements are usually recommended. In particular, they are critical if you have had a previous pregnancy affected by NTDs.

## IRON

Iron is a mineral essential for carrying oxygen around in the blood. Iron deficiency can lead to anemia. While some of the iron in our bodies is found in the hemoglobin molecule that carries oxygen around in our blood, the body also stores iron for future needs. Your iron needs increase significantly during pregnancy (to supply iron to your developing baby), so this is a time when the body draws on these iron stores. If you begin your pregnancy with good iron stores, you are less likely to become iron deficient. Iron-rich foods include lean red meat, eggs, legumes, tofu, whole grain breads and cereals, nuts, seeds and green leafy vegetables. The iron in plant foods (called non-heme iron) isn't as well absorbed as the iron in red meat, but absorption can be improved in the presence of vitamin C. Eating fresh salads, berries, kiwi or citrus fruits with most meals can help.

> Eating fresh salads, berries, kiwi or citrus fruits with most meals can help you absorb non-heme iron.

## VITAMIN D

Vitamin D is a fat-soluble vitamin produced in your skin during exposure to UV radiation from the sun. Having enough vitamin D while you are pregnant is important as your baby relies on your vitamin D stores, so making sure you have good levels when you conceive is essential. Low levels during pregnancy may affect the amount of calcium in your baby's bones. Unfortunately, vitamin D deficiency is on the rise because most of us spend too much time indoors, and we have been encouraged to protect our skin from the damaging effects of the sun when we are outdoors. There are only a few naturally occurring sources of vitamin D, including fatty fish (such as salmon and sardines), eggs, milk, cheese and butter. It is also added to margarines and, more recently, to some brands of milk and soy milk. In Chapter 4, we explain the safest way to expose your skin to the sun to optimize vitamin D levels.

## IODINE

Iodine is a naturally occurring mineral that is required by the thyroid to synthesize the thyroid hormones that regulate metabolism. In babies and young children, thyroid hormones play an important role in physical and mental development. A deficiency of iodine can lead to learning difficulties and affect physical development, particularly hearing. Starting your pregnancy with adequate stores of iodine is important. In fact, the American Thyroid Association recommends that all women who are pregnant, breastfeeding or considering pregnancy take a prenatal vitamin with iodine. The best food source of iodine is seafood. We also get iodine from other foods including milk and vegetables, but the amount varies depending on how these foods, are grown and processed. We also recommend that you purchase iodized salt, rather than ordinary salt or sea salt, and use sparingly in home cooking.

## WHAT YOU SHOULD AVOID

We have outlined what you should be eating, but there are also some foods you should stay clear of while trying to conceive. Apart from alcohol and caffeine (discussed on pages 15 and 17), there are a few other foods to consider avoiding or minimizing once you start preparing for pregnancy.

## HIGH MERCURY FISH

Fish is an important source of nutrients during pregnancy, including iodine and omega-3 fats, but some fish should be limited or avoided when you are pregnant or planning a pregnancy due to their higher content of mercury. Mercury is a heavy metal that occurs naturally in the environment and accumulates in the aquatic food chain, including fish. High levels of mercury can harm your unborn baby's developing nervous system, so it is a good idea to reduce your exposure to mercury before you become pregnant.

While all fish will contain some mercury, the levels in most fish and seafood do not pose a significant risk when consumed in moderation—the recommendation when pregnant is to limit fish intake to two to three servings (12 ounces total) per week. However, a few varieties of fish are particularly high in mercury, and these should be avoided if possible or limited. These include swordfish, shark, king mackerel, tilefish and bigeye or ahi (yellowfin) tuna. According to the Federal Food and Drug Administration, other varieties of fish, such as canned fish (including chunk light tuna), are low in mercury and can be safely eaten on a regular basis.

For more details visit americanpregnancy.org/pregnancyhealth/fish mercury.htm.

## LARGE AMOUNTS OF MEAT OR PROTEIN

Lean meat is a good source of iron, zinc, protein and vitamin $B_{12}$. But we recommend only moderate amounts. (There is no specific amount that is "too much," but we know that risk increases incrementally with increasing intake.) High intakes of red meat and processed meats may increase your risk of developing diabetes during pregnancy and type 2 diabetes later in life. Too much protein, including protein supplements, has also been linked to smaller babies, who suffer greater health problems at birth. Infertility and problems with ovulation may be less likely if you choose vegetable over animal protein.

This doesn't mean you need to avoid red meat altogether, but if you are a big meat eater, you might consider alternating it with plant proteins, including legumes (such as lentils, chickpeas and canned or dried beans) and tofu. If you do eat meat, choose lean cuts and avoid processed meats, which have been linked with cancer, diabetes and heart disease risk.

## TOO MANY EGGS

Eggs are a good source of protein, iron, zinc, vitamin $B_{12}$ and vitamin D. However, studies have found a relationship between high egg intake (more than seven eggs per week) and gestational diabetes risk. The high cholesterol content of eggs may be responsible.

This doesn't mean you should avoid eggs, because they are otherwise a nutritious and convenient protein source. But limiting your egg intake to less than one per day and alternating them with other protein sources is a good idea.

## TRANS FATS

Trans fats are produced in food processing through a process known as hydrogenation, used to improve the stability of vegetable oils and to convert liquid oils into solid fats. They are also created naturally by bacterial action in the gut of ruminant animals such as sheep, cattle and goats, and occur naturally in dairy products, beef, veal and lamb.

Trans fats are a type of fat that we should all avoid, as they worsen cholesterol levels and can increase heart disease risk. It is also important to reduce your intake if you are planning a pregnancy. One study found that eating more trans fats decreased the chances of getting pregnant due to problems with ovulation.

In the United States, the battle that public health advocates have been waging against trans fat seems to be working. A new report shows that since 2000, the level of trans fat in Americans' bloodstreams has dropped nearly 60 percent. This is in large part due to the fact that since January 2006, the Food and Drug Administration has required food manufacturers to list trans fat on Nutrition Facts labels. This makes it easy to identify and avoid foods high in these fats.

### SIX TIPS TO AVOID TRANS FATS

1.  Avoid deep-fried fast foods and takeout—takeout is more difficult in pregnancy as many of the "healthier" choices, such as salads, sandwiches, wraps and sushi, are off the menu due to food safety concerns. Alternative options include grilled fish, vegetable-based soups or stir-fries and tomato-based pasta.
2.  Avoid manufactured cookies and cakes unless they state that they are free of trans fats on the nutrition label—make your own healthy snacks instead (see the recipes in Part 5 for some ideas).

3. Avoid manufactured pies and pastries—try making homemade varieties using phyllo pastry or whole grain bread as a base.

4. If you eat margarine, choose one that is free of trans fatty acids—or use avocado, natural nut spreads or tahini instead.

5. If you eat meat and poultry, choose lean varieties or cut off any visible fat or skin before cooking.

6. Choose low-fat dairy products and limit use of cream and butter—low-fat evaporated milk makes a good cream alternative, and butter can be replaced with the alternative, spreads mentioned above.

## HIGH GI CARBS

High GI carbs are foods containing carbohydrates that are digested and absorbed quickly. Unfortunately, most breads and breakfast cereals (whether whole grain or not), rice (white or brown), potatoes, crispbreads, crackers and low-fat snacks are high GI. Soft drinks and candy such as jelly beans are also moderate to high GI. They raise blood glucose levels more than is desirable, forcing your body to secrete more insulin. Because all women become more and more insulin resistant as pregnancy progresses, there's a risk that your insulin-producing cells won't cope with the high demand, precipitating the common condition called gestational diabetes (we've devoted Chapter 7 to this topic). Although there's no proof yet that a high GI diet causes gestational diabetes, we think it's best to stay on the safe side and replace high GI carbs with low GI carbs. Your blood glucose is also the fuel for your baby's growth, and even moderately elevated blood glucose levels may cause your baby to gain excessive body fat, increasing his or her risk of childhood obesity. We've devoted another whole chapter (Chapter 6) to this important subject, focusing on the importance of exercise. And all the advice in Part 4 will help you choose the best sources of carbohydrates with a low GI—those that are slowly digested and absorbed—and full of dietary fiber, vitamins and minerals. You'll be pleased to know that most fruits and vegetables, legumes, pasta, oats, barley, quinoa and some brand-name breads and breakfast cereals are low GI.

## This for that—replacing high GI with low GI foods

Simply replacing high GI foods with low GI alternatives will give your overall diet a lower GI and deliver the benefits of low GI eating. Here's how you can put slow carbs to work by cutting back high GI foods and replacing them with alternatives that are just as tasty.

| IF YOU ARE CURRENTLY EATING THIS (HIGH GI) FOOD | CHOOSE THIS (LOW GI) ALTERNATIVE INSTEAD |
| --- | --- |
| Breads such as soft white or whole wheat; smooth textured breads, rolls, scones | Dense breads with whole grains, whole grain and stone-ground flours and sourdough |
| Breakfast cereals—most commercial, processed cereals including cornflakes, Rice Krispies, cereal bars | Traditional rolled oats, muesli and the commercial low GI brands listed in the table on page 109 |
| Cakes and pastries | Raisin bread and blueberry muffins may be healthier baked options; yogurts and low-fat puddings also make great snacks or desserts. |
| Candies | Chocolate is lower GI but high in fat; healthier options are raisins, dried apricots and other dried fruit. |
| Chips and other bagged snacks such as Doritos, pretzels, Cheez Doodles | Fresh grapes or cherries; dried fruit and nuts |
| Cookies | A slice of whole grain bread or toast with jam or fruit spread |
| Crackers | Crisp vegetable strips such as carrots, bell peppers or celery |
| French fries | Leave them out! Have salad or extra vegetables instead. Corn on the cob is a better takeout option. |
| Granola bars | Try a nut bar or dried fruit and nut mix. |
| Potatoes | Try sweet potatoes, new potatoes, or taro—or just replace with other low GI or non-starchy vegetables. |
| Rice, especially large servings of it in dishes such as risotto, nasi goreng, fried rice | Try basmati or Uncle Ben's Converted Rice, pearled barley, cracked wheat (bulgur), quinoa, pasta or noodles. |
| Soft drinks and fruit juice drinks | Try plain sparkling mineral water or seltzer with a slice of fresh lemon or lime. Fruit juice has a lower GI (but it is not a lower calorie option). Water is best. |
| Sugar | Moderate the quantity. Consider pure floral honey, apple juice and agave nectar as alternatives. |

## FOODS THAT POSE A MICROBIOLOGICAL RISK (FOOD SAFETY)

The risks associated with food poisoning really only come into play once you are pregnant, and we discuss this in more detail in Chapter 3. But as you won't know you are pregnant in the first few weeks, it is a good idea to become familiar with the high-risk foods. The main risk in pregnancy is infection with a bacteria called *Listeria monocytogenes*. While you are no more likely to be infected when pregnant, it can cause miscarriage or stillbirth if you are. For this reason it is recommended that all pregnant women avoid foods that are more likely to be contaminated. These include soft cheeses (such as brie, camembert and ricotta), unpasteurized dairy products, pâté, cold precooked chicken or meat, processed meats (such as ham and salami), raw or smoked seafood, soft-serve ice cream, and preprepared salads or fruit salads. You can also reduce your risk by being careful how you prepare foods at home: Always wash your hands before handling food; wash plates and utensils well between preparing raw and cooked foods; store cold or frozen foods correctly; and heat foods to the correct temperature when cooking, particularly meat and chicken.

Other risks include *Salmonella* bacteria, which contaminate the shells of most eggs and are still present in products that are not cooked, such as fresh mayonnaise (cooking will kill *Salmonella*). Bean sprouts are another *Salmonella* hazard. Toxoplasmosis is a condition that arises from eating uncooked or undercooked meat. It is also a risk if you have close contact with an infected cat, so get your partner to handle any kitty litter and make sure you wear gloves when gardening.

## LIVER

Liver is particularly high in vitamin A and eating it too regularly can cause high levels to build up in your body. High levels of vitamin A during pregnancy can cause birth defects. You should also avoid foods containing liver, such as pâté and liverwurst, because of the risk of listeriosis.

## TO SUPPLEMENT OR NOT TO SUPPLEMENT?

» **Folate** The U.S. Public Health Service recommends that all women who are trying to conceive should take a folic acid supplement for at least one month prior to becoming pregnant and for the first three months of their pregnancy. Folate is a B-group vitamin that has been shown to reduce the risk of your baby developing birth defects such as spina bifida. The usual recommendation for pregnancy is 400 to 800 micrograms per day, but women who are at higher risk (for example, if you have a family history of spina bifida or you have preexisting diabetes) are advised to take a higher dose (4 milligrams or 4,000 micrograms)—you should discuss this with your doctor.

» **Iodine** The American Thyroid Association recommends that all women who are pregnant, breastfeeding or considering pregnancy take an iodine supplement of 150 micrograms each day. Kelp and seaweed supplements are not recommended as they contain varying amounts of iodine. If you have an existing thyroid condition, you should talk to your doctor before taking a supplement.

» **Prenatal vitamin and mineral supplements** The benefits of folate supplementation in early pregnancy are clear, but the evidence for multivitamins is still lacking. The use of these supplements (without folate) has not been found to reduce the risk of birth defects, and when taken in addition to folate, they don't appear to provide additional benefits. However, prenatal vitamins are typically prescribed for women who are planning to become or are already pregnant, especially if they have any dietary restrictions or health problems or take medications that affect the absorption or use of particular nutrients. Since prenatal vitamins are specifically designed for pregnancy, they contain the recommended amount of folate needed to support a healthy pregnancy.

» **Vitamin A** Supplements should be strictly avoided during pregnancy and when trying to conceive, as large amounts of this vitamin can cause birth defects. It is best to obtain vitamin A from food during pregnancy, but if you do take a supplement, it is important that it doesn't provide more than 2,500 international units (IU) per day—if you take more than one supplement, calculate the

One of the main causes of male fertility problems is damaged sperm, which can occur as a result of oxidative stress. A recent review of the research found that couples undergoing assisted reproduction (for example, IVF) were more likely to become pregnant and have a live birth if the male partner took an antioxidant supplement. It is thought that antioxidants may improve sperm quality by reducing oxidative damage. A good balanced diet will contain plenty of antioxidants, but when it comes to nutrition, many males have a long way to go.

total vitamin A content and make sure it is less than this amount. Some acne and antiaging skin treatments contain vitamin A or related substances known as retinols or retinoids. These should also be avoided once you are trying to conceive, as the vitamin A in them can be absorbed through the skin into the bloodstream.

» **Herbal supplements** Herbal preparations are generally not recommended during pregnancy, as they have not been well enough studied to show that they are safe. Where possible, all herbal supplements should be avoided in the first trimester. If you are recommended a supplement when trying to conceive, it is important to ask about its safety during pregnancy and to avoid anything that has not been tested or proven to be safe in early pregnancy. In particular, laxative herbs, those which promote menstruation and those which have a stimulating effect on the uterus should be avoided. For further information, contact the National Center for Complementary and Alternative Medicine at (888) 644-6226 or visit nccam.nih.gov.

## WEIGHT MATTERS—SHOULD I WAIT?

If you're in the contemplation phase of planning a pregnancy, then now is a good time to assess whether you fall within the healthy weight zone, or should gain or lose a few pounds. (On page 64, we show you exactly how to assess your weight against your height.) You may be surprised or even shocked to learn that your pre-conception or starting weight in pregnancy has an enormous influence on your child's birth weight and future risk of diseases such as obesity and diabetes in childhood. One of the reasons that child obesity has become so prevalent is that both moms and dads are heavier than people were a generation ago.

Through mechanisms that we are only just beginning to understand, your child's metabolism and appetite are being "programmed" from the first days of pregnancy. If you're overweight, your baby will grow faster in the womb and after delivery. If you weigh less at the start of pregnancy, you will be more insulin sensitive, less likely to develop gestational diabetes and you will have a lighter baby with fewer complications at delivery.

If you want to become pregnant soon, you may not reach your ideal weight before you conceive, but losing even small to moderate amounts of weight can improve fertility and reduce pregnancy risks. Since losing weight can improve fertility and because women usually don't know they are pregnant in the first few weeks, it is important that your pre-conception weight-loss plan is not overly restrictive and contains all the nutrients needed in early pregnancy. Aiming for a gradual weight loss of no more than 1 pound per week is ideal. Once you do get pregnant, Chapter 4 shows you how to assess your weight and determine the optimal amount of weight to gain during pregnancy.

## LOSING WEIGHT SAFELY

Losing weight gradually and eating better rather than dieting may sound simple, but we know that for most people, losing weight and keeping it off is difficult. So how do you go about this? It starts with changing the way you think.

» **Don't think about going on a diet.** The only way to lose weight permanently is to change your eating habits and include some regular physical activity. The key is to make gradual changes that will fit in with your lifestyle and that you can continue for a lifetime.

» **Be patient and realistic.** Think about how long it took to put the weight on—you can't expect to lose it overnight. Also recognize that now is not the time for rapid weight loss and that focusing on the nutritional needs of you and your future baby needs to take priority.

» **Recognize the benefits.** Rather than thinking about the difficult aspects of weight loss and what you might need to give up, think about all the benefits that will come from eating well. Focus on getting your body in optimum shape to manage pregnancy and on providing your baby with the best possible start in life.

Focus on healthy eating habits, not dieting.

» **Learn to enjoy healthy food.** Think about food as nourishment for your body and your baby—to provide your baby with the best possible environment in which to develop, you will need to eat good quality food. Buy some healthy cookbooks or cooking magazines and experiment with new foods to find those that satisfy your appetite and taste buds.

» **Moderation is the key.** There is no need to totally avoid any foods if you enjoy them—all foods (apart from those which pose a food safety risk once you are pregnant) can be included as part of a healthy eating plan. Obviously, you need to set some limits, but cutting out all your favorite foods and feeling guilty about eating is not the way to go. Remember, your new eating plan needs to be for life. It should mean eating better, not less.

» **Balance food with regular exercise.** Losing weight isn't just about food—combining healthy eating habits with regular exercise is the best way to lose weight and keep it off. As we have already mentioned, being fit can also mean an easier pregnancy and can help to manage weight gain during pregnancy and reduce the risk of developing gestational diabetes. The type and amount of exercise you do may change from pre-conception to pregnancy and beyond, and we have given you lots of tips in Chapter 6.

## SUMMARY
# 8 steps to making a healthy baby

*Improving your own health before you conceive and providing a healthy environment for your unborn child can go a long way toward ensuring they have the best possible start in life. Aim to take these steps toward improving your health three to six months before conception:*

1. If you smoke, stop.
2. Limit alcohol and coffee.
3. Improve your eating habits.
4. Begin a regular exercise routine.
5. If you are overweight, improve your diet and activity level to achieve gradual weight loss.
6. Take folate and iodine supplements.
7. Review your medications (including nonprescription medications and supplements) with your doctor.
8. Make appointments for pre-pregnancy health checks.

# PART 2
# So now you are pregnant

*There's lots of well-intentioned advice about eating during pregnancy. You know your baby needs nutrients to grow and develop, and it's easy to see why you, too, need a good diet to stay healthy for the long haul. Indeed, nutrition is so critical to pregnancy that many embryos don't make it if critical nutrients are missing. If that's not reason enough, there's now irrefutable evidence that the quality of your diet during pregnancy also affects your child's future health, long after they leave the womb. In Part 2, we describe this new research, explain what to eat, what not to eat and why, emphasizing the importance of optimal weight gain, optimal blood glucose levels and the benefits of a low GI diet, as well as the lowdown on the best forms of exercise for a healthy pregnancy. Finally, because gestational diabetes is common, we also devote a chapter to the subject, explaining how and why it is treated and managed.*

# Chapter 3

# The best conceivable diet for pregnancy

In the past decade, researchers have found that a mother's diet during pregnancy directly alters or "imprints" her baby's genetic code (DNA), resulting in changes called "epigenetic" marks. This relatively new field of research delves into how and why genes are permanently altered by the environment in which the tiny embryo grows. These studies indicate that a mother programs her child's metabolism in both good and bad ways. A poor diet during pregnancy predisposes a child to developing obesity or diabetes when he or she is older. A good diet helps protect them. This gives us new reasons for eating well during pregnancy.

Eating for two means eating twice as healthily.

## NUTRITION NEEDS IN PREGNANCY

While being pregnant increases your nutritional needs, the amount of extra food needed is much less than you might expect. During the first trimester, your energy or calorie needs remain the same as they were before you became pregnant. In the second and third trimester, *in theory*, you need around 10 percent more energy. This equates to around 150 calories per day, or the equivalent of a large apple and a glass of skim milk. Despite this, your requirement for some nutrients, like iron, increases by more than 10 percent. This means that the key to getting all the nutrients that you and your developing baby need, without gaining excessive weight, is to choose quality over quantity. Choosing nutrient-dense foods—those that are packed with important vitamins and minerals—without overloading on calories is particularly crucial in pregnancy.

## THE TOP SIX NUTRIENTS FOR PREGNANCY

Whether or not you are pregnant, eating a balanced diet with a variety of foods from each of the major food groups each day will help to ensure your body is getting all of the nutrients it needs for good health. While an adequate intake of all essential nutrients is important for a healthy pregnancy, some play an absolutely critical role in ensuring the optimal health of your developing baby.

### FOLATE

Folate (or folic acid) is a B-group vitamin which is important for your baby's development during the early stages of pregnancy. Consuming enough folate in early pregnancy has been shown to reduce the risk of your baby developing birth defects called neural tube defects or NTDs (when the neural tube doesn't close properly), the most common being spina bifida. We discuss NTDs in more detail in Chapter 5. Consuming enough folate (through your diet and supplements) has been found to prevent seven out of ten cases of NTDs. It is recommended that women who are planning a pregnancy take a folic acid supplement providing at least 400 micrograms for one month before becoming pregnant and during the first three months of pregnancy (in addition to diet, to ensure the 600 micrograms requirement is met). If you have a family history of NTDs, you should speak to your doctor as higher doses of folate are recommended. It is also important to include plenty of folate in your diet. Foods rich in folate include green leafy vegetables (such as spinach, broccoli, cabbage and brussels sprouts), as well as legumes (such as lentils, chickpeas and dried beans), asparagus, avocado, nuts, oranges and wheat germ. In 1996, the FDA published regulations that require the addition of folic acid to enriched breads, cereals, flours and other grain products. This means that most breads and cereals you eat will provide a good source of folate. If you are choosing organic, be sure to check the label for vitamin content, as "free of additives" can sometimes apply to added nutrients.

The recommended daily intake (RDI) for folate is 400 micrograms for nonpregnant women, and this increases to 600 micrograms during pregnancy and 500 micrograms while breastfeeding. The following tips will help you to maximize your intake, but for more information on the folate content of foods, see our nutrient guide on page 207.

## 10 TIPS FOR INCREASING FOLATE

1. Use avocado as a spread on sandwiches instead of butter or margarine, and use peanut butter on toast in place of butter.
2. Add spinach and fresh green herbs to pasta.
3. Have an orange or freshly squeezed orange juice with breakfast each day.
4. Add broccoli, bok choy and peanuts or cashew nuts to stir-fries.
5. Snack on a handful of peanuts or hazelnuts—these two contain the most folate of all nuts.
6. Switch out your garden salad for a baby spinach, orange and walnut salad.
7. Combine crushed hazelnuts and chopped parsley with whole grain bread crumbs as a coating for meat or chicken.
8. Add legumes to soups, casseroles and curries.
9. Toss chickpeas into a stir-fry or salad.
10. Add wheat germ to smoothies or sprinkle on your breakfast cereal.

## IRON

Iron is another critically important micronutrient for pregnancy. Requirements increase significantly because your baby is stockpiling sufficient iron to last him or her through the first five to six months of life outside. Your recommended daily intake of iron increases from 18 milligrams per day in the nonpregnant state to 27 milligrams per day during pregnancy, so a concerted effort is needed to ensure that you get enough. Thankfully, your body becomes much more efficient at absorbing iron in pregnancy, so if you start with good stores and are careful to include plenty of iron-rich foods in your diet, you may be able to avoid needing a supplement. For many women, this much iron can be difficult to obtain from food alone, so most pregnancy supplements have extra iron added. Iron supplements have an unfortunate tendency to cause constipation, but you can reduce this by drinking lots of water and eating high-fiber foods such as whole grains, fruits, vegetables, nuts and seeds.

Foods rich in iron include lean red meat, legumes, poultry, fish, tofu, eggs, nuts, seeds, whole grain breads and cereals, green leafy vegetables and iron-fortified foods such as breakfast cereals. See the nutrient guide on page 207 for the iron content of typical servings of these foods. The iron in plant foods (called non-heme iron) is not as well absorbed as the heme iron in animal foods, but this can be improved by eating foods rich in vitamin C (such as citrus fruits, berries, kiwi, peppers and tomatoes) at the same meal. Tea and coffee may reduce iron absorption, so these are best drunk between rather than with meals. Calcium supplements can also reduce iron absorption, so they are best taken at a different time from your iron-rich meals.

## 10 TIPS FOR INCREASING IRON INTAKE AND ABSORPTION

1. If you eat meat, include lean red meat a few times per week.
2. On a vegetarian diet, eat a variety of iron-containing foods such as legumes, tofu, green leafy vegetables, nuts, seeds and whole grains (especially quinoa) regularly.
3. Snack on iron-rich foods such as a mixture of dried apricots, prunes and nuts; roasted chickpeas; or whole grain rye crackers with hummus.
4. Start your day with a whole grain cereal topped with a vitamin C–rich fruit such as berries or kiwi.
5. Add tomato or baby spinach to whole grain sandwiches for lunch to improve iron absorption from your bread.
6. Include legumes in soups and salads.
7. Choose whole grain pasta, brown rice, quinoa or barley in place of regular white rice and pasta.
8. Eggs are also a good source of iron and can be hard-boiled or scrambled for breakfast, or made into an omelet or frittata for a quick and easy meal.

9. Use nut spreads (such as almond, cashew or peanut butter) on toast in place of butter.
10. Homemade muffins containing dried fruit, nuts and whole wheat flour make a healthy iron-rich snack (see the recipe on page 280).

## OMEGA-3 FATS

Omega-3 fats are a form of dietary polyunsaturated fat that play many important roles in our body. There are three omega-3 fats in our diet that are considered essential, in that our body can't make them: alpha-linolenic acid (ALA), eicosapentaenoic acid (EPA) and docosahexaenoic acid (DHA). These fats, particularly DHA, are needed for your baby's brain, nerve and eye development, making them particularly important during pregnancy.

While adults have some ability to form the longer chain fats EPA and DHA from the shorter chain ALA, this ability appears to be limited in infants, who rely on their mother for DHA. Most of their stores are accumulated in the last trimester of pregnancy, so ensuring you have an adequate intake at this time (as well as while breastfeeding) is important. A higher intake of omega-3 fats may have other benefits for your child, too. One study found that women who ate three fish meals per week were less likely to have a premature baby. Another found that the children of women who had a higher intake of omega-3 fats during pregnancy were less likely to be obese at three years of age.

The main sources of omega-3 fats in our diet are oily fish but others include flaxseeds, chia seeds, flaxseed oil, walnuts, soy products, eggs and lean meats. Our nutrient guide on page 208 provides details of the omega-3 content of these foods. EPA and DHA are mainly found in fish and seafood while ALA is found in plant foods. There are also, now, a number of foods that have been fortified with omega-3 fats, from bread and cereals to yogurt and soy milks. The source of omega-3 in many of these products is the long-chain omega-3 fat DHA from algae, making them a good option for increasing intake of these important fats for vegetarians and those who don't eat fish or seafood. Examples include Stonyfield Yo Toddler organic yogurt, Tropicana Pure Premium Healthy Heart orange juice and Horizon Organic milk. If you don't include these foods in your diet regularly, it may be recommended that you take a fish oil supplement.

## 7 TIPS FOR BOOSTING OMEGA-3 INTAKE

1.  Include a serving of fatty fish (such as salmon, tuna, mackerel and sardines) at least once a week as well as other fish and seafood.
2.  Choose omega-3 eggs (produced by feeding hens a diet rich in omega-3 fats, usually from flaxseeds). They are easy to find in the supermarket as they are marked as "omega-3 enriched."
3.  If you don't eat fish, consider using foods which have been fortified with algal DHA, such as some yogurts (for example, Stonyfield's Yo Toddler).
4.  You could also take a fish oil or vegan DHA supplement— many prenatal vitamins contain fish oil.
5.  Use flaxseed oil as a salad dressing (you can't heat this oil, so don't use it for cooking).
6.  Use flaxseeds or chia seeds in baking bread and muffins, or sprinkle on cereal or in yogurt.
7.  Limit intake of trans fats (found mostly in fast foods and processed foods such as cookies and pastries) and omega-6 fats (such as oils and spreads made from sunflower, safflower or grapeseed), as these can prevent the short-chain omega-3 fats from being converted into the long-chain form that our body needs.

## CALCIUM

Calcium is important during pregnancy to maintain your own bone health and to provide enough calcium to form your baby's bones and teeth, particularly during the third trimester. If you don't eat enough calcium to meet these needs, your baby will draw calcium from your bones. Calcium needs are not increased during pregnancy because your body absorbs more from your diet. Nonetheless, many women don't consume enough of this important mineral in the first place, so pregnancy is a good time to improve your quota. You should aim for around 1,000 milligrams of calcium per day, which is the equivalent of three to four servings of a calcium-rich food each day. Pregnant teens will need extra calcium, aiming for 1,300 milligrams per day.

Good sources of calcium in the diet include milk, yogurt, cheese, calcium-fortified soy milk and yogurt, canned fish with bones (such as sardines and salmon), some green leafy vegetables (particularly Asian greens such as Chinese broccoli and bok choy, kale, collard greens and turnip greens), unhulled tahini (sesame seed paste), almonds, dried figs and tofu (particularly when set with calcium). For more details of the calcium content of these foods, see our nutrient guide on page 208.

## 10 TIPS FOR BOOSTING CALCIUM INTAKE

1. Include a fruit smoothie for snacks or a mug of hot milk before bed.
2. Have canned salmon on sandwiches or sardines on toast as a tasty breakfast or quick dinner (but don't pull out the bones!).
3. Make a calcium-rich stir-fry with tofu, Asian greens such as bok choy and Chinese broccoli and almonds.
4. Include green vegetables such as kale and broccoli with your meals regularly.
5. Snack on a handful of dried figs and almonds.
6. Use unhulled tahini paste as a spread, in making dips such as hummus or as a salad dressing.
7. Include a slice of cheese on toast, sandwiches or whole grain crackers.
8. Add yogurt to fruit for a tasty calcium-rich dessert.
9. Limit salt intake and caffeine intake, which can reduce the amount of calcium you absorb and retain in the body.
10. Ensure adequate vitamin D to help with calcium absorption (see page 47).

## IODINE

Iodine is a naturally occurring mineral that is needed by the thyroid gland in order to synthesize thyroxine, an important hormone that regulates metabolism. In babies and young children, thyroid hormones play a key role in physical and mental development. A deficiency of iodine can lead to learning difficulties and affect physical development and hearing.

The recommended daily intake for iodine is 150 micrograms for most adults, but this increases to 220 micrograms during pregnancy and 270 micrograms while breastfeeding, as your baby will take the iodine it needs from you. Though iodine deficiency is not typically a problem in the United States, as most table salt is enriched with iodine, the American Thyroid Association recommends that all women who are pregnant, breastfeeding or considering pregnancy take an iodine supplement of 150 micrograms each day. Kelp and seaweed supplements are not recommended as they contain varying amounts of iodine and can even cause toxicity (too much iodine). It's best to speak with your doctor before taking any iodine supplement, especially if you have a preexisting thyroid condition.

The best source of iodine in our diet is seafood. We also obtain iodine from vegetables, but the amount varies depending on how and where these foods are grown and processed. While we don't recommend that you add salt to your food, if you use it in cooking (for example, when boiling rice or pasta), it's best to buy iodized salt and use sparingly, particularly if you don't regularly consume other iodine-rich foods. Our nutrient guide on page 209 provides more detail on the iodine content of foods.

### 4 TIPS FOR INCREASING IODINE INTAKE

1. Include a few meals of fish or seafood each week (but avoid those which are not recommended in pregnancy—see later in this chapter, "Mercury in fish," page 53).
2. A glass of milk or container of yogurt with cereal or as a snack will provide iodine as well as calcium and other nutrients.

3. If you use salt in cooking or on your meals, choose iodized salt rather than other types.
4. Sushi is a good way to get iodine, but for food safety reasons needs to be homemade, without raw fish, and eaten fresh. Nori (sushi wrappers) can also be chopped into salads and stir-fries for vegetarians or non-fish eaters, but avoid kelp, which can contain very large amounts of iodine.

## VITAMIN D

Vitamin D is a fat-soluble vitamin produced in your skin during exposure to UV radiation from the sun. It has long been known to play an important role in bone health, helping calcium to be absorbed from the gut and into the bones, but more recent research has found that its role is far more widespread than just bone health. In fact low levels have been associated with an increased risk of colon cancer, schizophrenia, diabetes, multiple sclerosis and heart disease. Unfortunately, vitamin D deficiency is on the rise because we all spend more time indoors and try to protect our skin from the damaging effects of the sun when outdoors. A recent Australian study found that 41 percent of pregnant women with gestational diabetes had low levels of vitamin D.

Having enough vitamin D during pregnancy is especially important because your baby relies directly on your vitamin D stores. Having ample amounts before conception is ideal, but you can still make good when the deed is done. Vitamin D is important for your baby's developing bones, and low levels during pregnancy may affect the amount of calcium in your baby's bones. A severe deficiency causes a deformity of the bones called rickets, a condition that used to be quite common in countries that have long winters.

It is difficult to obtain all your vitamin D needs from food alone. There are only a few naturally occurring sources, including fatty fish (such as salmon and sardines), eggs, milk, cheese and butter. Vitamin D is also added to margarines and (more recently) is included in some brands of milk and soy milk. Our nutrient guide on page 209 provides details of the vitamin D content of these foods. It is recommended that most children and adults under fifty years of age consume 15 micrograms per day, including during pregnancy and while breastfeeding. The shortfall is obtained by exposing some skin to the sun at safe times of the day (see box below).

## Safe sun exposure

While we get some vitamin D from food, the best source is UVB radiation from the sun. Vitamin D forms in the skin when it is exposed to UV from sunlight, but the amount will depend on your location, the time of the year, the time of the day and cloud cover.

During summer, most of us can maintain adequate vitamin D levels by exposing our face, arms and hands (or an equivalent area of skin) to a few minutes of exposure to sunlight outside the peak UV periods (10 AM to 3 PM) on most days of the week. Those with darker skin may need longer exposure.

Source: ods.od.nih.gov/factsheets/VitaminD-HealthProfessional

## 7 TIPS FOR BOOSTING VITAMIN D INTAKE

1. For a cooked breakfast have scrambled eggs on toast.
2. Include canned salmon or tuna or a hard-boiled egg on sandwiches or in salads at lunch.
3. Salmon frittata or quiche makes a vitamin D–rich lunch or light dinner.
4. Replace sausages or hamburgers on the barbecue with salmon patties or fresh salmon, tuna or mackerel steaks.
5. Add salmon or tuna to pasta and rice dishes.
6. Try a salmon and baby spinach omelet for a healthy and tasty weekend breakfast or quick evening meal.
7. Consider choosing a fortified milk such as Horizon Organic or a fortified soy milk such as Silk or ZenSoy.

## TO SUPPLEMENT OR NOT?

The only supplements that are routinely recommended in pregnancy are folate and iodine. As discussed earlier in this chapter, it can be difficult to get the amounts needed for pregnancy from food alone, and the U.S. Public Health Service and the American Thyroid Association recommend that all pregnant women take them in supplement form. If you have low levels of vitamin D, then you will need a supplement to boost your intake, and if you don't eat fish, then taking a fish oil or vegetarian DHA supplement will help to ensure you have enough of these important fats while you are pregnant. Some women will also need an iron supplement if they are unable to maintain adequate iron levels from diet alone.

Whether taking other vitamin and mineral supplements is beneficial is unclear, although there is some evidence that taking a multivitamin and mineral supplement containing folate can reduce the risk of birth defects. If you do supplement, it is important that you don't take large amounts of any vitamins or minerals that may be unsafe in pregnancy, particularly vitamin A (see page 54). The best option is a specially formulated prenatal vitamin and mineral preparation that contains a balanced amount of the vitamins and minerals needed in pregnancy including those above, without anything you shouldn't be taking. These supplements vary in their content, so it is best to check with your doctor, midwife or dietitian about which is the best option for you.

## WHY FOOD SAFETY MATTERS

Food poisoning is unpleasant for anyone, but when you are pregnant it can be more serious—for both you and your unborn baby. Since the hormone changes in pregnancy can inhibit your immune system and make it more difficult to fight infections, taking care to prevent foodborne illness is particularly important.

To reduce your risks of all types of foodborne illness, focus on freshly cooked foods and well-washed, freshly prepared fruit and vegetables. Leftovers can be eaten if they are refrigerated promptly and kept no longer than a day.

These are the biggest risks during pregnancy:

» **Listeriosis** is a serious infection caused by the *Listeria* bacteria, which are found naturally in some foods. It can take up to six weeks for symptoms to occur and if the infection passes on to your unborn baby, it can cause miscarriage or stillbirth. The good news is that careful preparation, handling and storage of foods, as well as avoiding high-risk foods, can minimize the chances of infection. High-risk foods include soft cheeses, cold processed meats, cold cooked chicken, raw seafood, prepared salads and fruit salads, pâté, soft-serve ice cream and unpasteurized dairy products.

» **Salmonellosis** is caused by the *Salmonella* bacteria, with the usual symptoms including nausea, vomiting, abdominal cramps, diarrhea, fever and headache. You are no more likely to develop this while pregnant, but in rare cases, it may cause miscarriage. High-risk foods include raw eggs, undercooked meat and chicken and any type of salad sprouts (including alfalfa, broccoli, onion, sunflower, clover, radish, snow pea, mung bean and soybean), whether or not they are cooked.

» **Toxoplasmosis** is uncommon but if you are infected during pregnancy it may lead to brain damage or blindness in your unborn child. Undercooked meats, unpasteurized goat's milk and unwashed fruit and vegetables are the main food risks, particularly if your cat likes to use your vegetable garden as a toilet. Toxoplasmosis is more commonly caused by touching cat and dog feces when cleaning up after your pet, or by touching contaminated soil in the garden. Being pregnant is a good excuse to hand over the kitty litter duties to your partner! If you garden, always wear gloves and make sure you wash your hands well afterwards. Washing thoroughly after touching any animal is a good move.

## Food safety tips

» Keep cold food refrigerated (below 40°F/5°C) and hot food steaming hot (above 140°F/60°C) before serving. This will stop the growth of food poisoning bacteria.

- » Separate raw and cooked food, and don't use the same utensils, such as cutting boards and knives, for both.
- » Wooden cutting boards are fine for fruit and vegetables, but a plastic board is best for meat and eggs.
- » Defrost frozen food in the fridge or on the "defrost" setting in the microwave, never at room temperature.
- » Keep utensils, cutting boards and your kitchen countertops and sink clean.
- » Cook food thoroughly. Cook poultry and ground meats until well done, right through to the center. No pink should be left visible and all juices should be clear.
- » Always wash and dry your hands thoroughly before and after handling food.
- » Prepare food as close as possible to when you are going to eat it.
- » Refrigerate leftovers as soon as the food stops steaming, and if you cook large amounts of food to store, divide it into smaller portions or shallow containers before putting it into the fridge or freezer. Make sure there is good air circulation around the containers.

## FREQUENTLY ASKED QUESTIONS

**"My husband has a family history of food allergies. Should I avoid certain foods in pregnancy to reduce the risk of allergies for our child?"**

The American Academy of Pediatrics does not recommend restricted diets during pregnancy as there is no evidence that they reduce the risk of your child developing an allergy, and have been associated with poor weight gain in babies. The same goes while breastfeeding. The only thing we know that can reduce the risk is to avoid smoking during pregnancy (and around the child once born) and to breastfeed if possible until six months of age.

## AVOID HARM

So far, we have focused on what you should eat, but there are also some foods and fluids that are best avoided or limited when you are pregnant, breastfeeding or trying to conceive.

## CAFFEINE

While small amounts of caffeine are believed to be safe during pregnancy, large amounts may increase the risk of miscarriage and premature birth. Remember that caffeine isn't only found in coffee but also in tea, energy drinks, cola drinks and chocolate. It is recommended that pregnant women limit their intake to 200 mg of caffeine each day. The table below gives a guide to the caffeine content of a variety of drinks and foods; however, it is important to realize that when it comes to coffee, these values are only approximate and can vary widely depending on how the coffee is made, the types of beans used and quantity consumed. An Australian study looking at the amount of caffeine in close to one hundred espresso coffees purchased from different outlets found a wide variation in caffeine content ranging from 25 to 214 mg. A more recent UK study similarly found a sixfold difference in the caffeine content of espresso coffees, ranging from 51 to 332 mg. So if you enjoy espresso-style coffee, it is probably best to limit your intake to no more than one per day when pregnant, and to choose smaller size drinks containing a single shot of espresso.

## CAFFEINE CONTENT OF COMMON DRINKS AND CHOCOLATE*

| FOOD OR DRINK | SERVING SIZE | CAFFEINE CONTENT (MG) |
|---|---|---|
| Coffee, brewed | 8 oz cup | 95–200 |
| Coffee, instant | 8 oz cup | 27–173 |
| Coffee, espresso (the basis of café-style coffees such as cappuccino, latte, etc.) | 1 oz (1 shot) | 40–75 |
| Cocoa powder (for chocolate-flavored milk and baking) | 1 tbsp | 8 |
| Chocolate, dark | 1.45-oz bar | 41 |
| Chocolate, milk | 1 oz | 1–15 |
| Formulated caffeinated beverages or energy drinks | 8 oz | 47–80 |
| Tea | 8 oz | 14–61 |
| Cola soft drink | 12 oz | 0–55 |

* Values vary for individual products.
Sources: mayoclinic.com/health/caffeine/AN01211 and fda.gov/downloads/Drugs/Resources
ForYou/Consumers/BuyingUsingMedicineSafely/UnderstandingOver-the-counterMedicines
/UCM205286.pdf

## ALCOHOL

There is no safe level of alcohol consumption during pregnancy and the American Pregnancy Association recommends that it is best not to drink during pregnancy. If you are drinking heavily during pregnancy, your baby could be born with a condition known as fetal alcohol syndrome, which results in slow growth before and after birth and mental disabilities. Even drinking moderate amounts (one or two glasses a day) while you are pregnant may harm your unborn baby, possibly causing learning disabilities, mental retardation, behavioral problems and poor growth. The risk of miscarriage and stillbirth are also increased. We recommend that you stay on the safe side and avoid alcohol completely. If you think your drinking may be a problem, then there's lots of help available, starting with your doctor.

## MERCURY IN FISH

Fish is a good source of protein and other minerals, low in saturated fat and the best source of omega-3 fats and iodine in our diet—as discussed earlier, these nutrients are particularly important in pregnancy. It's therefore a good idea to include fish in your diet regularly while pregnant and breastfeeding, but you need to be careful about which fish you choose. Mercury occurs naturally in the environment and accumulates in the aquatic food chain, including fish. Some fish contain higher levels of mercury and may harm your unborn baby or a young child's developing nervous system.

While all fish will contain some mercury, the levels in most seafoods do not pose a significant risk when consumed in moderation. The recommendation when pregnant is to limit fish intake to two to three servings (12 ounces total) per week. However, some varieties of fish are particularly high in mercury and these are best avoided—they include swordfish, shark, king mackerel, tilefish and bigeye or ahi tuna. According to the Food and Drug Administration, other varieties of fish, including canned fish, are low in mercury and can be safely eaten on a regular basis (that is, up to 12 ounces, or two average meals, per week). For more details visit www .fda.gov/Food/FoodSafety/Product-SpecificInformation/Seafood /FoodbornePathogensContaminants/Methylmercury/ucm115662.htm.

There is no need to panic if you have had the occasional meal of higher mercury fish—it is only when you eat these fish regularly that mercury levels can build up in the blood and cause problems for your unborn baby.

## VITAMIN A

Supplements of this vitamin should be avoided during pregnancy and when trying to conceive, as large amounts can cause birth defects. It is best to obtain vitamin A from food during pregnancy but if you do take a supplement, it is important that it doesn't provide more than 750 mcg per day—if you take more than one supplement, the total vitamin A content should be less than this amount. Daily intake of liver and other organ meats is not a good idea, either, because they are extremely rich sources of vitamin A. Some skin treatments contain vitamin A or related chemicals, known as retinols or retinoids, and these should also be avoided as the vitamin A in them can be absorbed through the skin into the bloodstream.

## HERBAL SUPPLEMENTS

We do not recommend herbal supplements during pregnancy as they have not been well studied to show that they are safe. Where possible, all herbal supplements should be avoided in the first trimester. While herbs are natural foods, concentrated forms of these foods are not. If you are recommended a supplement when trying to conceive, it is important to exercise a high level of caution. In particular, laxative herbs, those which promote menstruation and those which have a stimulating effect on the uterus may harm your unborn baby. For further information contact the National Center for Complementary and Alternative Medicine at (888) 644-6226 or visit nccam.nih.gov/health/supplements/wiseuse.htm.

## SMOKING, DRUGS AND OTHER HAZARDOUS CHEMICALS

In Chapter 1 we explained why avoiding smoking, recreational drugs and hazardous chemicals is important while you are trying to conceive, and this is even more critical once you are pregnant. Smoking during pregnancy increases the risk of miscarriage, ectopic pregnancy (implantation outside the uterus), premature birth and stillbirth. If you smoke, or if you are exposed to secondhand smoke from your partner (or others), your baby is more likely to have a low birth weight and has a higher risk of birth defects and sudden infant death syndrome (SIDS). Smoking during pregnancy may also increase the chances of your child being overweight later in life and increase their risk of developing hyperactivity (attention deficit hyperactivity disorder or ADHD). When it comes to recreational drugs, these may also harm your baby, and there is no safe level of use in pregnancy. If you are still smoking or using drugs when you become pregnant, quitting should be your number one goal—see "Three ways to quit" on page 15 for details on where you can get help. As mentioned on page 16 in Chapter 1, we also suggest using natural household cleaning agents and avoiding exposure to lead-based paints, herbicides and pesticides while pregnant.

## DEALING WITH COMMON PROBLEMS

Despite being a happy and exciting time, not everything about pregnancy is pleasant. Nausea, vomiting, constipation, heartburn and food cravings are all part and parcel of pregnancy for most women. While you may not be able to avoid these common complaints, having strategies to deal with them, if and when they arise, can help you cope.

### MORNING SICKNESS

Nausea and vomiting are almost universal during the first trimester of pregnancy and usually improve by the 12-week mark. In rare cases, they may continue until your baby is born. The exact cause is unknown, but pregnancy hormones are the likely culprit. While an unfortunate part of pregnancy, you can be assured that it doesn't cause any harm to your baby, unless it is severe enough to cause dehydration and weight loss. Although it is usually referred to as "morning sickness," it can occur at any time of the day—and if you are unlucky, it may stick around all day!

If you are experiencing nausea and vomiting, the following suggestions may help:

» Try a piece of dry toast or dry crackers before getting out of bed—you might want to keep a supply of dry crackers by your bed.

- » Eat small regular meals and snacks over the day rather than three large meals.
- » Eat according to your appetite; don't worry about normal mealtimes.
- » Avoid strong smelling foods, and, if possible, see if someone else can help with cooking and preparing your meals.
- » Get plenty of fresh air and keep rooms well ventilated.
- » Drink plenty of fluid. If you can't tolerate plain water, try ginger ale, lemonade or mineral water. You may find it better to sip on fluids over the day rather than large amounts at a time.
- » Avoid fatty and highly spiced food.
- » Try eating foods or drinks containing ginger, such as ginger tea or flat ginger ale, which some studies have found may help with nausea in pregnancy.
- » If you are vomiting, it is important to take extra care to stay hydrated. Oral rehydration solutions or diluted soft drinks may be useful.

## When nausea and vomiting become too much

A small number of pregnant women (fewer than 1 in 100) will experience severe nausea and vomiting; they are unable to keep down food and fluids, resulting in weight loss and dehydration. In medical speak, this is called hyperemesis gravidarum. If this happens, you need to seek medical attention. Treatment commonly involves hospital admission so you can be given fluids via an IV and medication to stop the vomiting.

## HEARTBURN

Heartburn, or indigestion, is a common problem in the second half of pregnancy as your baby grows and puts pressure on your stomach. It feels like "heartburn" because the strong mix of food, acid and enzymes is pushed back into your esophagus, irritating the lining that is not normally exposed to acid in this way. While you can't remove the cause, there are some things you can do which may help:
- » Eat small frequent meals throughout the day.
- » Drink between meals rather than with meals.
- » Avoid spicy or fatty foods.
- » Leave at least two hours after a meal before you go to bed or lie down.

» Eat slowly and always sit down to eat; avoid eating on the run.

» Relax at mealtimes and try not to eat when you are stressed or upset.

» Avoid coffee—including decaffeinated coffee. Tea may be a better choice for people with heartburn.

» Sleep with an extra pillow, or elevate the head of your bed using a brick or block of wood.

» If none of the above help, talk to your doctor about an over-the-counter antacid that is safe to use in pregnancy.

## CONSTIPATION

Constipation is not uncommon during pregnancy and is more likely to occur or be worse if you take an iron supplement. Increasing the fiber in your diet, drinking plenty of fluids and exercising regularly will usually help.

Good sources of fiber include whole grain breads and cereals, grains (such as barley, brown rice and quinoa), legumes, nuts, seeds, fruit and vegetables. You could also try a couple teaspoons of psyllium husks mixed into cereal, yogurt or a glass of water or juice. Make sure you drink plenty of water along with the psyllium as it works by absorbing water to make your stools softer and easier to pass. If you take it without adequate fluid, it can have the opposite effect and make constipation worse. If you can't tolerate this, you could try a fiber supplement such as Metamucil™ or Benefiber™.

If these changes don't help and your constipation is bothering you, speak with your doctor or midwife. Most laxatives and laxative herbs are not recommended during pregnancy, so it is important to get advice about what is safe to take.

## FOOD CRAVINGS AND AVERSIONS

We don't know why, but around eight out of ten women will experience cravings for at least one particular food while pregnant. It may be for something sweet, salty or spicy—and possibly even foods that you wouldn't usually eat. Many women also experience aversions to some foods, often things that they previously ate and enjoyed. You may even find that the smell of some foods becomes unbearable. Nature works in strange ways!

In most cases it is fine to satisfy your cravings, as long as the foods you crave are not those which should be avoided in pregnancy (for example, due to food safety concerns) and you don't eat them to the exclusion of more nutritious foods. It is important to continue to eat a balanced diet. Some women find that they have a desire to eat things that are not food, such as dirt, clay, chalk or even laundry detergent! This could be harmful to both you and your baby and should be avoided. There is some evidence that this could be due to iron deficiency, so if you have unusual cravings, speak to your doctor.

## TIPS FOR DEALING WITH CRAVINGS AND AVERSIONS

1. If you are craving a food that you shouldn't eat during pregnancy, try to find an alternative that will still satisfy your taste buds—for example, canned salmon in place of smoked salmon, cream cheese in place of ricotta, or yogurt in place of soft-serve ice cream.

2. If your cravings are less than healthy ones, indulge in small amounts of your craved food but make sure you continue to eat a variety of healthy meals and snacks. You could also try to find some healthier options—for example, hot chocolate made with low-fat milk (rather than a chocolate bar) or some roasted chickpeas (in place of potato chips).

3. If you can't face your usual plate of steamed vegetables at dinner, try a cold salad of roasted vegetables or make them into a blended soup.

4. Not eating meat? Make sure you still get enough protein and iron by substituting other protein sources—try tofu in a stir-fry, lentil bolognese, bean tacos or a chickpea curry.

5. If the smell of food cooking turns you off your meal, try to get someone else to help with food preparation and cooking, and try cold meals such as sandwiches and salads.

## HEALTHY EATING CHECKLIST

Having read this chapter, it might be helpful to make a note of everything you eat and drink over one week to see at a glance where you could increase your intake of these important nutrients. Try to include quantities and types of food and drink, cooking methods, brands and sauces. Eat normally so you can see a clear picture of what you consume over an average week.

# EXAMPLE DAY

|  | **EXAMPLE DAY** |
|---|---|
| Breakfast | ½ All-Bran® <br> 1 cup whole milk <br> 1 slice whole wheat toast <br> 1 teaspoon butter |
| Morning snack | ½ container Yoplait Original French Vanilla Yogurt <br> Apple—1 medium |
| Lunch | Chicken, avocado & veggie whole wheat sandwich <br> (1 whole wheat roll, 3½ ounces chicken breast, 2 lettuce leaves, 1 tomato, ½ English cucumber, ¼ avocado) |
| Afternoon snack | 100% whole grain bread—2 slices, toasted <br> Hummus—½ teaspoon <br> Coca-Cola Zero—8 ounces |
| Dinner | Grilled steak—7 ounces <br> Baked potato—with 2 teaspoons sour cream <br> Carrot—1 medium, steamed <br> Peas—½ cup, steamed <br> Water—16 ounces <br> Tangerine—1 large |
| Evening snack | 8 rice crackers <br> Low-fat cheddar cheese—1 slice |
| Other (e.g., supplements, physical activity) | Walking—30 minutes |
| Caffeine | |
| Alcohol | |
| Other drinks | |

Make seven copies of the blank table on next page and complete with everything you eat and drink each day for seven days.

# FOOD RECORD

| | DAY | DATE |
|---|---|---|
| Breakfast | | |
| Morning snack | | |
| Lunch | | |
| Afternoon snack | | |
| Dinner | | |
| Evening snack | | |
| Other (e.g., supplements, physical activity) | | |
| Caffeine | | |
| Alcohol | | |
| Other drinks | | |

# Chapter 4

# Ideal weight gain

This chapter doesn't beat around the bush. Pregnancy is a time when many women gain more than enough. Traditionally, dietary advice for pregnancy has focused on making sure there's adequate intake of all the essential nutrients (as you learned in Chapter 3). That's not surprising, considering the fact that the requirements for many nutrients are higher than at any other time in life. Unfortunately, weight gain during pregnancy, despite its importance, is not given the emphasis that it deserves. In this chapter, we show you how to calculate your ideal weight gain (depending on your height and pre-pregnancy weight), and how to monitor and keep it under your control.

As a routine part of care, many obstetric care providers will keep an eye on your weight gain, but most will steer away from discussing it for fear of causing embarrassment or needless anxiety. Women will often discuss the subject among themselves, especially if it's faster and greater than they expected. Many will tell you that even after the birth, they retained a few pounds, and found them difficult to budge. While their experience is common, we want to assure you that weight gain during pregnancy *is* under your control and, indeed, it's good practice for you to monitor it yourself, so that you gain the ideal, or optimal, amount.

Okay, so what's ideal? The optimal amount of weight gain over pregnancy is one that results in a "desirable pregnancy outcome." That means a healthy baby, born at full term (about forty weeks, or nine months plus one week, gestation) with a birth weight of 6–9 pounds. In women from affluent countries like the United States, who start pregnancy weighing 140–160 pounds, the average weight gain over pregnancy is about 28 pounds, and the average infant birth weight is 7 pounds, 8 ounces. But these are averages only. You'll be pleased to hear that there's a range of weight gains that are considered ideal. The desired amount depends to a large extent on your pre-pregnant weight. For a woman who is underweight, a higher weight gain is desirable, while an overweight mom should gain less.

Of increasing concern, the average weight gain during pregnancy has increased over the past few decades. From the 1940s to the 1960s, weight gain tended to hover around 22 pounds. The recommendation to all pregnant women at the time, irrespective of their starting weight, was to restrict their weight gain to just 15 pounds. This advice stemmed largely from the observation that increased weight gain was directly related to higher birth weight, and higher risk of pregnancy complications. In 1970, however, the Institute of Medicine (IOM) determined that restriction of weight gain during pregnancy was likely to be harmful, and the weight gain recommendations were eased to a range of 20–26 pounds. Nonetheless, by 1980, the average weight gain in American women had increased to 33 pounds. In the US, up to 40 percent of women gain more weight than is recommended during pregnancy. The increase has occurred in women of all shapes and sizes, including the slimmest and the heaviest, with far-reaching consequences.

## WHY DOES WEIGHT AND WEIGHT GAIN MATTER?

Weight gain in pregnancy is an excellent predictor of the baby's weight at birth. This, in turn, predicts how well your baby copes in the first days and months of life. That's the reason for the proud tradition of announcing not only the baby's sex but its birth weight as well. Like many things in life, however, there is a happy medium. If you gain too little, it can mean a small baby who has been born too lean with little body fat. Small babies, defined as those born weighing less than 5 pounds, 8 ounces, have a higher chance of having poor outcomes during and after birth. Paradoxically, they are more likely to become overweight as adults and have a greater risk of high blood pressure and heart disease. On the other hand, a baby that grows too big or too fast also has poor outcomes. Excessive weight gain during pregnancy and high birth weight (greater than 9 pounds) are both linked to complications at birth, such as emergency Caesarean delivery, fetal macrosomia (a baby having excess fat), physical injury and postpartum hemorrhage. Just as importantly, excess weight gain also predicts the future health of both mother and baby. In the long run, excessive weight gain in pregnancy has contributed to the current epidemic of obesity in women and children. A woman who gains too much during pregnancy gives birth to an overweight daughter, who in turn is more likely to be an overweight child and young adult, who is then more likely to gain excessive weight during her first pregnancy and give birth to a child with excess fat, and the cycle repeats itself.

## Body fat in babies—the studies

The most concerning aspect of excessive weight gain in pregnancy is the body fat of the baby. The Southampton Women's Study in the UK found that almost half the children in the study were born to women who gained excessive weight during pregnancy, resulting in greater body fat mass at birth, as well as at four years of age and again at six years of age. In contrast, appropriate pregnancy weight gain as defined by the IOM was linked to lower levels of fat in the children. In Sweden, a study of nearly 150,000 male army recruits found that their BMI (body mass index) at eighteen years of age was directly linked to their mother's pregnancy weight gain—but *only* if their mother had been overweight or obese at the start of pregnancy. If she was normal weight, her pregnancy weight gain did not predict her son's future BMI.

Excessive weight gain also worsens the mom's state of insulin resistance, which is an otherwise normal physiological adaptation to pregnancy. However, in excess, insulin resistance has adverse effects on blood fats and on other metabolic markers, including blood glucose levels, blood pressure and inflammatory factors.

## RECOMMENDED GUIDELINES FOR WEIGHT GAIN

In 1990, the IOM established the first set of guidelines for weight gain in pregnancy. In 2009, these guidelines were updated to take into account the larger number of women who entered pregnancy with excess body fat. The new recommendations are shown in the box on the next page. Most developed countries around the world use these guidelines.

## IOM Guidelines for Pregnancy Weight Gain 2009

**THE BMI HERE REFERS TO YOUR BMI AT THE START OF PREGNANCY**

| | |
|---|---|
| BMI less than 18.5 (underweight) | 28–40 pounds |
| BMI 18.5–24.9 (normal weight) | 25–35 pounds |
| BMI 25–29.9 (overweight) | 15–25 pounds |
| BMI 30 or greater (obese) | 11–20 pounds |

## HOW TO CALCULATE YOUR BMI

Your BMI is a rough guide to your body fat mass relative to your height. To calculate yours, you need to know your pre-pregnancy weight in pounds without clothing and your height in inches without shoes.

$$\text{BMI} = \text{weight (pounds) divided by}$$
$$\text{the } \textit{square} \text{ of your height in inches (that is, height squared)}$$
$$\text{multiplied by 703}$$

An example:

If your weight is 140 pounds and your height is 64 inches,
then your BMI is $(140 / [64 \times 64]) \times 703 = 24$

## RATE OF WEIGHT GAIN

Your rate of weight gain (that is, pounds per week) over the course of pregnancy varies according to trimester. Very little is usually gained in the first trimester. Indeed, the developing embryo weighs only .04 ounces and is not quite three-quarters of an inch long at eight weeks of age: It's about the size of a bean. During those first critical weeks and months, the rapidly multiplying cells have differentiated into various tissues and tiny organs, which is why the *quality* of the diet, not the *quantity*, is so important at this stage. From 12 weeks onward, however, you can expect to gain steadily at a rate of about ¾ to 1 pound until the baby is delivered at around 40 weeks gestation (38–42 weeks is considered within the range of normal gestation).

It is interesting to look at the makeup of the pregnancy weight gain. Much of it is water (about 60 percent), 30 percent is fat and only 8 percent is protein. For a woman who gains the typical 28 pounds, about 5–10 pounds represents a natural increase in her own fat stores. Your blood volume also increases, as does the weight of your uterus and breast tissue. The baby weighs on average 6½ to 8½ pounds at birth and the placenta that is delivered after the baby weighs about 1½ pounds.* The components of pregnancy weight gain are shown in the box below.

Not surprisingly, the biggest variation among different women is in the amount of fat stored. It ranges from no increase at all in some developing countries to 11 pounds or more in affluent countries.

## Components of Weight Gain in Pregancy (in pounds)

| | |
|---|---|
| **RESULTS OF CONCEPTION** | **11** |
| Baby | 7.7 |
| Amniotic fluid | 1.8 |
| Placenta | 1.5 |
| **MATERNAL TISSUES** | **9.4** |
| Water | 3.7 |
| Uterus and breasts | 3.1 |
| Blood | 2.6 |
| **FAT STORES** | **7.1** |
| **TOTAL WEIGHT GAIN** | **27.5** |

Using the figures in the box, we can calculate that about 70,000 additional calories are needed to grow these new tissues over a period of about nine months, equivalent to roughly 240 calories per day. An average woman normally eats about 2,100 calories per day, so the extra 240 calories is about 10 percent above pre-pregnant needs. But interestingly, careful studies in well-nourished women reveal either no change in energy intake during pregnancy or only a minor increase, so small that it simply can't explain all the extra energy deposited in new tissues. Scientists have long been puzzled

---

* The placenta is the organ that connects the baby to the wall of the uterus to allow nutrient uptake, waste collection and gas exchange via the mother's blood supply.

# Avoiding excess weight gain—the research

Reducing excessive weight in pregnant women is only now being given the research attention that it deserves. The question is how best to optimize weight gain (not too much, not too little). Because of concerns about birth defects, weight loss medications and supplements such as appetite suppressants clearly have no place. But simplistic instructions to restrict food intake could result in inadequate intake of essential micronutrients. Taken too literally, food restriction could increase the risk of low-birth-weight babies or of babies with developmental abnormalities.

It would be logical to expect that general advice about a healthy diet and physical activity during pregnancy is helpful in limiting weight gain and excess growth of the baby. Unfortunately, when put to the test, that approach has shown disappointing results. One-on-one sessions with a dietitian do improve nutritional intake, but it's not clear whether it reins in excessive pregnancy weight gain. One study of 400 overweight women in Finland found no differences in weight gain in those who were given individualized advice by a dietitian versus those who were given "usual care" by a GP or midwife-nurse.

Some studies have specifically examined whether it's helpful for overweight pregnant women to follow a calorie-restricted diet, as they would if they were trying to lose weight. These studies reported that there was a significant reduction in the mother's weekly weight gain (in fact as much as a half a pound less per week in one study), but the effect on the baby's birth weight was highly variable from study to study. Some studies found no difference; another study found a very large reduction in the baby's birth weight, on the order of one pound. In another, there was a trend for women in the lifestyle advice group to have a larger baby! The most encouraging study showed that a much more intensive intervention consisting of ten one-hour consultations with a trained dietitian halved the amount of weight gain (compared with usual care) in obese pregnant women.

Interestingly, one Australian study found that overweight women given a personalized weight goal at the beginning of pregnancy and instructions to just weigh themselves at regular intervals (no advice on diet) gained less weight than those given usual care during pregnancy. Unfortunately, this advice was not effective among the women with a BMI above 35 (that is, those who were obese and therefore needed it most).

The most recent review of the medical literature found that on the whole, diet and physical activity interventions were effective in reducing pregnancy weight gain. Thus, while simplistic lifestyle advice (eat less, exercise more) is not likely to be effective, a well-planned program of focused dietary counseling sessions by trained individuals is worthwhile. The Academy of Nutrition and Dietetics website (eatright.org) provides a search function that allows you to find dietitians who consult in your area.

as to why this is so. Some suspect that physical activity declines and others suspect that absorption of nutrients increases, but at the present time, we really don't know why most women do not appear to eat more energy during pregnancy. So much for the old saying "eating for two"!

## THE BEST DIET FOR OPTIMIZING PREGNANCY WEIGHT GAIN

At the present time, we believe that low GI diets are the healthiest and safest diets for optimizing pregnancy weight gain. In nonpregnant overweight and obese women, low GI diets are linked to improved sense of fullness, greater weight and body fat loss and a better capacity to prevent weight regain after a large weight loss. It is therefore reasonable to expect that low GI diets might help prevent excess pregnancy weight gain. This proved to be the case in a recent study in 800 Irish women (the ROLO Study) who were at risk of delivering overly large babies. Those instructed to follow a low GI diet gained significantly less weight during pregnancy than those given no dietary advice. Importantly, this study showed that a low GI diet significantly reduced the risk of developing glucose intolerance during the third trimester, a potential harbinger of type 2 diabetes later in life.

> A low GI diet may reduce the risk of giving birth to a
> large baby without increasing the risk of a small baby.

Dr. John Clapp III, a Californian obstetrician, found that a low GI diet that was initiated at around 12 weeks gestation reduced both weight gain and birth weight in a small group of women. The six women allocated the higher GI diet gained an average of 44 pounds compared with only 26½ pounds in the low GI group.

Although more research is needed, low GI diets might also improve glucose metabolism during pregnancy. Remember, pregnancy can be likened to a metabolic stress test. Low GI diets reduce the levels of insulin in the blood after meals and also improve insulin sensitivity in people with type 2 diabetes. Higher insulin sensitivity is likely to reduce the chance of excess weight gain. In fact, high insulin concentrations in the mother's blood are linked to greater weight gain during pregnancy and a greater tendency to retain the weight after pregnancy. While increasing insulin resistance in pregnancy is a normal physiological consequence of pregnancy, in excess it can cause impaired glucose tolerance and gestational diabetes.

## Food supplements and pregnancy weight gain

Many studies have examined whether food supplementation (for example, milk powders and other supplement drinks) during pregnancy is helpful or not, particularly in undernourished women with a low BMI. Food supplements containing calories and protein in normal proportions were found to increase total pregnancy weight gain and increase the birth weight of the baby. Importantly, the food supplements reduced the chances of having a small baby (under 5 pounds, 8 ounces) and perhaps the chance of premature delivery. When the mothers were followed up with later, supplemented mothers were the same weight as unsupplemented mothers, and there were no differences in the children's heights, BMI or body fat levels as teenagers. If your BMI is in the underweight range (see the box on page 71), consult your doctor about whether you may need a food supplement.

### High-protein diets and supplements

Some studies have specifically examined the efficacy of high-protein supplements. A large trial in Harlem, New York, found that adding daily protein shakes did not increase the mother's weight gain or the infant's birth weight. Indeed, there was a tendency for the babies to be born lighter (the opposite of the investigators' expectations) and an increased risk of stillbirth.

Similarly, some trials have looked at whether a high-protein diet (as opposed to high-protein supplements) is beneficial. They found a small increase in weekly weight gain and birth weight, but unfortunately, there may have been an increased risk of having a small baby, too.

To sum up, health authorities believe there's no justification for prescribing high-protein supplements to pregnant women. Not only do these products lack evidence of benefits, they may even be harmful. This applies to both undernourished and well-nourished women. Even in overweight women, who may be gaining weight too fast, there is nothing to suggest that they are helpful, and there may even be a small chance that they may limit the growth of your developing baby.

# 4

# steps to optimizing your pregnancy weight gain

**1** Work out your pre-pregnancy body mass index (BMI)

**2** Circle your current BMI range

**3** Circle your optimum weight in the first trimester

**4** Weigh yourself week by week throughout the second and third trimesters

We strongly recommend that you monitor your weight gain starting with the confirmation of your pregnancy or (if that's too late) with your first prenatal visit at around 12 to 13 weeks gestation.

The amount of weight you should gain when you are pregnant will depend on your weight when you conceive.

Work out your pre-pregnancy body mass index (BMI) by dividing your weight (in pounds) by your height (in inches) squared and multiplying the result by 703.

$$\text{BMI} = \left( \frac{\text{Weight in pounds}}{[\text{Height in inches}]^2} \right) \times 703$$

If you google "calculate BMI," you'll find numerous sites that do the math for you. If you don't recall your pre-pregnancy weight precisely, don't worry, a rough estimate will do. If you're in the first 13 weeks of pregnancy, you can safely guess your pre-pregnancy weight by subtracting 2 to 4 pounds from your current weight. If you feel you've gained weight more quickly, subtract 10 pounds from your current weight.

An example:
If your weight is 165 pounds and your height is 67 inches (5'7"), then your BMI is (165/[67 × 67]) × 703 =26

**Your pre-pregnancy weight =** \_\_\_\_ **pounds**

**Your current height =** \_\_\_\_ **inches**

**Your BMI =** \_\_\_\_

**STEP 2**

Circle your current BMI range and the optimum weight gain range from the categories below, and then write this range in the bottom right-hand box of the chart in Appendix 1, page 295.

**BMI less than 18.5**    **Optimum weight gain range: 28–40 pounds**
**BMI 18.5–24.9**    **Optimum weight gain range: 25–35 pounds**
**BMI 25–29.9**    **Optimum weight gain range: 15–25 pounds**
**BMI greater than 30**    **Optimum weight gain range: 11–20 pounds**

**Note:** These figures are only for women expecting one baby—if you are carrying twins or more, then you will need to gain more weight than this. For all women, these are only guidelines, and you should always follow the recommendations of your pregnancy health-care team.

**STEP 3**

In the chart below, circle your optimum weight gain in the first trimester and then your optimal rate of weight gain per week in the second and third trimester.

| PRE-PREGNANCY BMI | TOTAL WEIGHT GAIN POUNDS | WEIGHT GAIN IN 1ST TRIMESTER POUNDS (TOTAL) | WEIGHT GAIN IN 2ND AND 3RD TRIMESTER POUNDS PER WEEK |
|---|---|---|---|
| less than 18.5 (underweight) | 28–40 | 1.2–4.5 | 1.2–1.5 |
| 18.5–24.9 (normal weight) | 25–35 | 1.2–4.5 | 0.9–1.2 |
| 25.0–29.9 (overweight) | 15–25 | 1.2–4.5 | 0.5–0.7 |
| greater than or equal to 30.0 (obese) | 11–20 | 1.2–4.5 | 0.5–0.7 |

Week by week throughout the second and third trimester, weigh yourself once per week at the same time of day and insert your new weight in the chart at the back of this book (see Appendix 1, pages 294–95). If you find yourself gaining too much, then take heed and try to eat smaller portions. If you are concerned, talk to your doctor and consider consulting a registered dietitian (see eatright.org).

## FREQUENTLY ASKED QUESTIONS

**"Is it safe to lose weight during pregnancy?"**

In most cases it is not recommended that you intentionally lose weight during pregnancy. Restricting your diet to lose weight may mean that you and your baby don't get enough of the nutrients needed during pregnancy. However, if you started your pregnancy overweight, it is safe to gain less weight than a woman who conceived at a normal weight. See the guidelines on page 71 to determine the amount of weight gain you should aim for.

**"I'm having twins—how much weight should I gain?"**

If you are carrying twins, you should naturally expect to gain a bit more weight than women who are having just one baby. The IOM recommends a total weight gain of 37–54 pounds for women who are at a healthy weight at the time of conception (a BMI of less than 25), 31–50 pounds for women who are overweight (a BMI of 25–30) and 25–42 pounds for women who are obese (a BMI of 30 or more). Of course, these are general guidelines and you should always follow the recommendations of your obstetric-care provider.

## Chapter 5

# Blood glucose levels in pregnancy

Pregnancy is a time when carbohydrates and the glycemic index (GI) are of special relevance. This is because your average blood glucose level throughout the day, whether it's low, moderate or high, is directly correlated with the baby's growth rate in utero. Quite simply, glucose is the primary fuel for your baby's growth. We've known this fact for a long time and it's the main reason why women who have type 1 diabetes (a condition that requires daily insulin injections to maintain normal glucose levels) are given intensive medical attention before and during a pregnancy. It's also the principal reason why pregnant women are routinely tested in pregnancy to determine if they have developed gestational diabetes (see Chapter 7 for more on this).

Your blood glucose fuels your baby's growth.

## WHY YOUR BLOOD GLUCOSE LEVELS MATTER

Even if you are healthy and well, if your glucose levels are too low, your baby's growth might be too slow for its own good. Conversely, if your blood glucose levels tend to be on the high side, your baby will grow rapidly and become too big for its own good (not to mention yours!). An overly large baby is linked to greater risk of delivery complications for both mother and child. These infants have an increased risk of childhood obesity, as well as higher risk of metabolic diseases such as diabetes and hypertension in adulthood. As usual, moderation is a good thing.

One of the reasons we wrote this book is because infant birth weights and childhood obesity have increased hand in hand over recent decades in most industrialized nations. We now know that life inside the womb (in utero) is a critical period for the metabolic programming of obesity in later life. The mother's weight at the time of conception and weight gain from early to late pregnancy profoundly influences infant birth weight (as we described in Chapter 4). But we believe that the increasing GI of the modern diet might also be a factor.

Pregnancy is a very real metabolic stress test. Even during the first trimester, your baby draws so much glucose from your bloodstream that your fasting glucose levels and day-long levels are lower (by about 9 mg/dl) than they are in the nonpregnant state. Pregnant women use carbohydrates at a greater rate at rest and during exercise than do non-pregnant women. Thus, one of the first metabolic adaptations your body makes to pregnancy is a greater capacity to produce glucose in the liver (this is called gluconeogenesis). This makes perfect sense because it means that even if your access to food is temporarily restricted, your growing baby will still be getting the energy it needs.

Pregnancy produces quite profound metabolic changes in all women and these become more evident as pregnancy progresses. Insulin secretion in response to eating doubles between the first and third trimesters, and insulin resistance increases by about 50 percent. This seems to be a normal physiological adaptation. Scientists believe that the higher degree of insulin resistance, particularly in the muscle mass, helps to redirect glucose away from mother's muscle cells toward her baby, enhancing its growth and eventual survival outside the womb.

Plasma glucose levels in the baby always mirror those in the mother, with a difference of about 10 mg/dl in favor of the mother. This difference increases as the pregnancy progresses. The mother's insulin cannot cross the placenta, but from about 12 weeks of age onward, the baby makes its own.

Insulin is often described as a "master hormone," the conductor in charge of orchestrating many biochemical pathways in the body. In particular, we know it's an anabolic hormone that stimulates growth and buildup of new tissues. Scientists believe that high blood glucose levels in the mother give rise to high levels in the placenta and umbilical cord blood, which in turn stimulates enlargement of the baby's insulin-producing cells (called beta cells) and the secretion of excess insulin. This extra dose of insulin is the direct cause of above normal rates of growth.

## Smaller babies are also at risk

Smaller babies or babies born prematurely (or those small for their gestational age) also have an increased risk of developing metabolic problems later in life. They have smaller or fewer beta cells (the insulin-producing cells) in their pancreas and are more likely to develop type 2 diabetes as adults.

Thus, optimizing the glucose environment of your baby may reduce the tendency to metabolic problems later in life. Sustained reductions in food intake will lower your glucose levels and therefore reduce your baby's rate of growth and final birth weight. On the other hand, if your blood glucose levels are running high for most of the day, this can lead to excessive growth and increased risk of giving birth to a large baby. In fact, women with undiagnosed diabetes during pregnancy are five times more likely to have a baby with a birth weight greater than 9 pounds. It is also clear that efforts to reduce blood glucose levels in mothers with diabetes, including dietary strategies, will curb excessive growth and reduce the likelihood of having a complicated delivery. Studies in women with diabetes suggest that reducing their average blood glucose levels to less than 130 mg/dl will prevent the birth of a large baby. In healthy pregnant women, researchers have found a link between the blood glucose concentration one hour after a meal and the baby's body fat level, as determined by ultrasound measurements. Merely reducing this spike in blood glucose (for example, by adopting a low GI diet) may, therefore, help control your baby's growth.

Unfortunately, relatively little research has been carried out to define the optimal range of blood glucose levels that results in a good pregnancy outcome in women who don't have diabetes. To help answer this question, a large observational study was recently conducted in nine countries including the United States involving 23,000 pregnant volunteers. They underwent a 75-gram glucose tolerance test (a kind of surrogate meal test) at the same stage of pregnancy, and all were followed up with at delivery. The findings were astounding. The higher the blood glucose levels in the fasting state, or at one hour or two hours after the glucose drink, the higher the number of infants born above the 90th percentile for birth weight (that is, larger than nine out of ten babies), and the higher the number of adverse pregnancy outcomes (such as an emergency Caesarean delivery).

Some studies suggest that blood glucose levels in healthy women without diabetes program the offspring's growth even after birth. Monitoring a group of 263 healthy pregnant American women, researchers found that their average blood glucose level at the end of the second trimester directly predicted their child's body mass index at three years of age.

The most common way to reduce blood glucose levels in women with diabetes who are pregnant is by restricting the amount of carbohydrates in the diet. That's not surprising, because carbohydrates are the main determinant of the rise in blood glucose after meals. However, in healthy women without diabetes, reducing carbohydrate intake and substituting protein in place of carbohydrates may have undesirable consequences (see Chapter 4). One review of high-protein supplements and diets indicated that this strategy increased the number of small babies born weighing 5 pounds, 8 ounces, or less. High-protein diets, particularly those high in red meat and eggs, have also been linked with higher chances of developing gestational diabetes.

## CARBOHYDRATES AND THEIR GI

While the amount of dietary carbohydrates is clearly a major determinant of the rise in blood glucose after eating, in practice, most people tend to eat much the same amount of carbohydrates from day to day and meal to meal. This makes the type of carbohydrate, particularly the glycemic index, or GI, of the carbohydrate food, an important consideration. Some foods, such as legumes and milk, naturally contain carbohydrates that are digested more slowly and have less impact on blood glucose. These foods are called low GI foods, and a low GI diet is one in which the meals are associated with lower blood glucose peaks after eating. On the other hand, a majority of modern starchy foods, including most breads and breakfast cereals, potatoes and rices and even many processed whole grain foods, are rapidly digested and absorbed, and produce a high blood glucose peak or "glycemic spike." Sweets made with glucose, such as jelly beans and regular soft drinks, also have a relatively high GI. But surprisingly, many foods containing added sugars, such as ice cream, yogurt and chocolate, produce a relatively lower glucose response.

You can't guess the GI of a food by its appearance, ingredients or nutrient composition—it has to be tested in real human subjects who consume the food under highly standardized conditions. Professor

David Jenkins and his colleagues at the University of Toronto developed and perfected the GI methodology, allowing us to classify all carbohydrate foods on a simple scale of 0 to 100, according to their glycemic impact. While the GI was considered controversial for some years, low GI diets are now recommended by various diabetes associations around the world. We now know the GI of about 2,500 different products, including most of the important carbohydrate sources in our diet. You can access a free searchable GI database at glycemicindex.com as well as in the annually updated *Low GI Shopper's Guide to GI Values*. You may also want to subscribe to the electronic *GI News* newsletter to read the most recent findings from around the world (ginews.blogspot.com).

Using the GI is easy. You don't need to remember numbers or do any math. You simply swap your usual bread, breakfast cereal, rice or snack for a lower GI one (this for that). You just need to know which ones are low GI. In Part 4 of this book, we show you how to incorporate low GI foods in a healthy balanced diet for pregnancy.

Using the GI is easy. You don't need to remember numbers or do any math. You simply swap your usual bread, breakfast cereal, rice or snack for a lower GI one (this for that).

## WHY USE THE GI IN PREGNANCY?

Nearly twenty-five years ago, an obstetrician in England wondered whether dietary fiber could be used to reduce excessive blood glucose levels without restricting carbohydrates in the diet of his pregnant patients. He studied 15 normal healthy pregnant women who ate three different diets for two weeks each, in random order. He found that the typical Western diet, with 40 percent carbs and only 10 grams of fiber, was associated with increasing insulin resistance and higher glucose levels. In contrast, when the women consumed the two high-fiber diets (one with 40 percent carbs and one with 60 percent carbs), their insulin sensitivity remained unchanged and their glucose metabolism improved.

However, very high-fiber diets are not for everyone, and the *type* of fiber may be more important than the total amount. Blood glucose levels after eating can be reduced by simply slowing down the rate at which the carbohydrates are digested and absorbed. Soluble viscous fiber such as that found in legumes, barley and oats can slow digestion, but insoluble fiber such as wheat bran makes no difference, even in large amounts. When it comes to digestion, differences in the physical and chemical architecture of the starch and sugars present in a food appear to be much more important than fiber content. Many carbohydrate staples, such as rice, bread and potatoes, contain fully hydrated and gelatinized starch, making them easy to digest and consequently high GI. Indeed, the typical diet has a moderate to high GI, depending on the proportions of starchy foods versus fruit and dairy products.

In 2006, we published one of the first studies in the world in which the GI was applied to pregnancy. More than 60 healthy pregnant women living in Wollongong, NSW, were assigned to either a low GI diet or a conventional healthy high-fiber diet for the second and third trimesters of pregnancy. On average, they were overweight, but some were normal weight and others obese. All women saw the research dietitian five times during the course of their pregnancy and were given instructions and encouragement to follow the diet to which they were allocated. The findings were nothing short of astounding. Infants born to the women following the low GI diet were significantly lighter, and had a lower percentage of body fat, compared with the babies of mothers following the conventional diet. More importantly, the women following the low GI diet were *ten times* less likely to deliver a large baby (greater than the 90th percentile of that time), suggesting that a low GI diet could also reduce the chances of childhood obesity. Women assigned to the low GI diet found it just as enjoyable, affordable and acceptable to all members of the family as those following the conventional high-fiber diet.

In our Wollongong study, women on the low GI diet were more likely to report that the diet was "easy to follow."

Dr. John Clapp III, the Californian obstetrician mentioned in Chapter 4, studied a low GI diet in pregnancy. He took a group of 12 healthy pregnant women and instructed them to consume a low GI diet for the first trimester of pregnancy, and then assigned them to either a high GI or a low GI diet for the remainder of pregnancy. The women who ate the high GI diet showed progressively higher post-meal glucose levels, whereas those who ate the low GI diet remained the same. Remarkably, the women who consumed the high GI diet all delivered a very large infant with a mean birth weight 2 pounds, 3 ounces heavier than the infants born to women who ate the low GI diet. The women who ate the high GI diet also gained significantly more weight during pregnancy.

There is one study that suggests that a poor diet, even if low GI, has undesirable outcomes in pregnancy. Dr. Theresa Scholl and her colleagues from the University of Medicine & Dentistry of New Jersey conducted an observational study of more than 1,000 pregnant women living in an underprivileged area in New Jersey. None of the women received dietary instruction, and they consumed on average 50 percent of their carbohydrates from refined sugars. They found that those who self-selected a low GI diet gave birth to infants who were 3.5 ounces lighter, but they also had a bigger chance of delivering an underweight baby weighing less than 5 pounds, 8 ounces. Smaller babies, like very large babies, experience more complications in the early months of life, and are at greater risk of metabolic diseases such as heart disease in later life. Scholl's study indicates that it's important to incorporate *healthy* low GI foods into your pregnancy diet and not focus on the GI alone. Don't worry—in Part 4, we show you how it's done.

## DOES A LOW GI DIET REDUCE YOUR CHANCE OF DEVELOPING GESTATIONAL DIABETES?

It is conceivable that adopting a healthy low GI diet early in pregnancy might reduce the risk of developing gestational diabetes. If you start off with a higher weight and/or gain weight too quickly, you are at greater risk of being diagnosed with the condition when you are tested with the 75-gram glucose tolerance test during pregnancy. One observational study, also from Wollongong, found that women who developed gestational diabetes were eating fewer low GI foods than those who did not develop the condition. However, to date, there are too few studies to guide us, and these have an insufficient number of participants to make a firm recommendation. To help answer the question, we are presently conducting a large randomized controlled trial to test the hypothesis that a low GI diet reduces the risk of developing diabetes in pregnancy. But based on the weight of evidence available right now, we can say that the use of a healthy low GI diet has no disadvantages and may offer some advantages, including higher insulin sensitivity, lower post-meal glucose levels and a reduction in excessive body fat in the baby.

## CAN A LOW GI DIET REDUCE THE RISK OF BIRTH DEFECTS?

Moderation is a good thing and that applies to glucose levels in the blood. Very high glucose levels are toxic to cells. That's why people with diabetes not properly controlled by diet or medications develop complications such as blindness, kidney failure, nerve damage and cardiovascular disease. High glucose levels are also implicated as one of the causes of the birth defect called a neural tube defect or NTD.

An NTD is an opening in the spinal cord or brain that should have closed during development. Normally, in the second week of pregnancy, specialized cells begin to fuse and form the neural tube. By week four, the neural tube closes, but if it does not close up completely, an NTD develops. In some instances, the brain and/or spinal cord are exposed at birth through a defect in the skull or vertebrae (back bones), a condition known as spina bifida. NTDs are one of the most common serious birth defects.

As we saw in Chapter 3, foremost among the causes of NTD is a relative deficiency of the vitamin folic acid, which is why folic acid supplements are routinely recommended for pregnancy. Diabetes, a condition characterized by high blood glucose levels if not properly managed, is also associated with a having a higher risk of a baby with NTD. For this reason, a woman with type 1 diabetes who is planning to have a baby should do her best to ensure she has optimal glucose control before she conceives.

The concern is well justified because of the known toxic effects of excess glucose in the blood of the mother on the embryo. At this early stage, the embryo has no beta cells and is unable to secrete insulin or regulate its own glucose levels. Studies have confirmed that markedly elevated glucose concentrations contribute to the development of birth defects.

In 2003, researchers from the March of Dimes hypothesized that women who had a higher intake of sugars or a higher glycemic index diet would have an elevated risk of having a pregnancy affected by NTD. To find out, they examined data from a large population study. More than 700,000 births, miscarriages and stillbirths, of which 653 were confirmed as NTD, were included. These cases were matched to a control infant randomly selected from hospital records. The investigators conducted in-person dietary interviews with the mothers, asking them to recall their diet from three months before to three months after conception. The findings were startling. They found that mothers whose diets had a high GI were more likely to have been overweight at the start of pregnancy and more likely to have had a baby with an NTD. If the women had a high BMI (greater than 30) *and* a higher GI diet, they were four to five times more likely to have given birth to a baby with an NTD. The effect was still present when mothers with a history of diabetes were excluded. They also found a relationship between higher sucrose content of the diet and NTD, but this included sucrose from all sources, including fruit and fruit juice. A study like this does not prove a cause and effect, but rather hints at a link that requires further research.

## SUMMARY: THE GI AND PREGNANCY

Although more research is still needed, the GI seems to be particularly relevant to pregnancy. Your baby's growth in the womb is directly related to your average blood glucose levels. This applies to perfectly healthy pregnant women as well as those who have developed gestational diabetes, which we cover in Chapter 7. It is possible that a healthy low GI diet will reduce your risk of having a large baby, especially if your glucose tolerance is worsening as your pregnancy proceeds. It may help to prevent excessive weight gain in pregnancy and reduce your chances of developing gestational diabetes. These are important outcomes, because they are relevant to your own and your child's future risk of obesity and chronic disease. The good news is that a healthy low GI diet is absolutely safe in pregnancy and doesn't require a great deal of discipline and sacrifice. You don't need to cut out whole food groups or specific foods (such as bread or sugar) or, indeed, any of your favorite foods. It is a delicious and easy diet to follow, as we show you in Part 4 of this book.

# Chapter 6

# Exercise in pregnancy

Sorry ladies, being "with child" is no longer considered a "confinement," an illness, or a time to put your feet up. It is a natural physiological state just like growth in children. Indeed, we now know that being physically *inactive* during pregnancy can be detrimental. Yet most women still have plenty of questions about appropriate exercise at this time. In this chapter, we explain the types of exercises that are best; how long, how hard and how often you should work out; and the precautions needed. Because every pregnancy is different, we advise all women to discuss their exercise plans with their doctor. If you developed diabetes or hypertension before pregnancy, or you have had a previous pregnancy in which there were complications (for example, a premature baby or pre-eclampsia), you should seek an individualized exercise program from a registered health-care professional. Even if you're perfectly healthy, it's a good idea to discuss your exercise plans at your first prenatal visit.

There are many specific benefits to staying active while you are pregnant, including optimal weight gain, improved mood and maintenance of your pre-pregnancy fitness level (see the box on the next page). If you work out regularly, your infant is less likely to accumulate excessive body fat and have weight problems as a child. In a study involving over 80,000 Danish infants, women who exercised during pregnancy for more than five hours per week had much less chance of giving birth to a large baby (more than 9 pounds), and they were no more likely to have a small baby. Exercise also reduced the risk of preterm birth. If you exercise regularly, there's also a reduced chance of developing gestational diabetes. If gestational diabetes does eventuate (see Chapter 7), then exercise will be an important part of your management plan.

## The benefits of exercise

Some of the benefits of exercising regularly throughout your pregnancy include:

- A general sense of well-being
- Less weight gain, less fat deposited
- Lower risk of cardiovascular complications
- Reduced risk of gestational diabetes
- Stress relief
- Improved posture
- Stronger back muscles, which can help manage back pain as your belly grows
- Improved sleep and management of insomnia
- Faster return to pre-pregnancy fitness and healthy weight
- Increased ability to cope with the physical demands of motherhood

Being fit will also help your body to cope better with the physical demands of pregnancy, labor and delivery. In the past, doctors were concerned that exercise might compromise the baby's growth, but recent research has made it clear that any risks are minimal compared with the enormous benefits to be gained. If you're healthy and not into exercise already, now's the perfect time to start the daily habits and discipline that should last a lifetime. Walking and swimming are both good ways to begin. Start slowly: Try 10 minutes for the first week, building up to 20 minutes and then to 30 minutes on most days of the week by the third week.

According to the American College of Obstetricians and Gynecologists guidelines, healthy women who have an uncomplicated pregnancy can continue their previous exercise habits after consultation with their doctor. It is also safe to start an exercise program during pregnancy, and regular exercise should continue after the baby is born, so you're setting a good example for the whole family. If you're an elite athlete, with your doctor's permission, you can continue to train during pregnancy, but not at the same intensity or duration. Some women may find it hard to accept that pregnancy and birth will interrupt sporting aspirations, but you can take heart from the fact that motherhood may actually enhance your future performance.

## HOW MUCH EXERCISE ARE YOU GETTING?

Your aim should be about six hours per week of moderate exercise (perceived effort 3 out of 10) or three hours per week of vigorous exercise (perceived effort 6 out of 10).

If you are doing a mixture of moderate and vigorous exercise, you can double your vigorous hours and add them to your moderate to determine your overall total. Use the chart below to record your current activity levels.

| ACTIVITY | MODERATE MINUTES PER WEEK | VIGOROUS MINUTES PER WEEK |
|---|---|---|
| DEDICATED TO EXERCISE | | |
| Gym (the treadmill, exercise bike) | | |
| Walking | | |
| Jogging | | |
| Cycling | | |
| Weights (or other resistance exercise) | | |
| Yoga, Pilates, etc. | | |
| JUST FOR FUN | | |
| Hiking | | |
| Tennis | | |
| Dancing | | |
| Gardening | | |
| Kicking a ball with the kids | | |
| Other | | |
| INCIDENTAL/OBLIGATORY ACTIVITY | | |
| Housework/cleaning | | |
| Laundry and ironing | | |
| Toddler care | | |
| Taking the stairs | | |
| Mowing the lawn | | |
| Cleaning the pool | | |
| Other | | |
| TOTAL | | |

## YOUR CHANGING SHAPE

Your changing shape and physiology, not just increasing weight, affect your physical abilities. As your pregnancy progresses, there are changes in weight distribution and body shape that cause your body's center of gravity to move forward and the normal curvature of the spine to increase. This makes some activities uncomfortable (such as jogging), and one in two women develop some degree of back pain. These changes can also alter your balance and coordination, particularly in the third trimester. In theory, you are more likely to fall, so activities that require good balance or involve a rapid change in direction are not recommended (such as rollerblading). Your higher weight also magnifies the forces across joints in the hips and knees. In weight-bearing exercise, such as running, the forces are 100 percent higher, increasing the risk of damage to susceptible joints.

## LOOSENING OF THE LIGAMENTS

During pregnancy, your joints will gradually loosen under the influence of the hormone (appropriately named) relaxin. This prepares the pelvic joints for birth, resulting in a heightened risk of injuries (such as strains and sprains). It is always important to listen to your body and not to overdo it. Care should be taken with any activity that involves jumping; jerky movements; frequent stopping, starting or changes of direction; and excessive stretching. Strengthening exercises are helpful, especially core strength exercises, but precautions are needed, as we explain later in this chapter.

## PHYSIOLOGICAL CHANGES

Your resting heart rate increases by 10–15 beats per minute during the second and third trimesters of pregnancy, and your maximum heart rate decreases. For this reason, you shouldn't use the normal target heart rates to determine exercise intensity during this time. It's best to use ratings of perceived exertion such as the Borg Rating of Perceived Exertion Scale shown on page 91. During the second trimester, the blood vessels that supply the placenta grow and multiply, and cause your blood pressure to fall. From the fourth month onward, your blood pressure will be 5–10 points lower than prior to pregnancy, and you may find yourself feeling dizzy when you rapidly change position, such as moving from lying down to standing up, or stopping suddenly. Leg exercises done lying on your back are best avoided because the weight of the baby can slow down the return of blood to your heart. You might like to do them lying on your side instead. For the same reason, long periods of standing still should be avoided.

The good news is that as pregnancy progresses, the body's ability to transport oxygen improves. Although the concentration of hemoglobin is lower during pregnancy, your hemoglobin levels might go up because of the increase in blood volume in order to meet the needs of your growing baby. Because oxygen requirements are increased, the lung volume on each breath increases. But the work of breathing becomes a little harder because of the pressure of the enlarged uterus on the diaphragm. This all means that there may be less oxygen available for exercising muscles during pregnancy. So don't be surprised to find that exercise feels harder and, indeed, your maximum exercise performance is reduced.

## OVERHEATING

During pregnancy, a major concern is your ability to dissipate the excess heat generated by exercise. Even at rest, your metabolic rate and, therefore, heat production is 10–20 percent higher than in the nonpregnant state. During exercise, your body temperature will rise in direct relation to the intensity of the exercise. Even if you exercise at a moderate pace in a pleasant climate, your core body temperature rises by 3°F/1.5°C after 30 minutes. If you work out in hot, humid conditions or at very high intensity, your ability to dissipate the extra heat can be compromised. During prolonged, strenuous exercise (for example, aerobics for more than 45 minutes), sweat loss and dehydration may interfere with your ability to regulate body temperature. In the worst-case scenario, your core temperature might continue to rise.

So what's the big deal? There are theoretical concerns associated with overheating, or hyperthermia, and the possibility that prolonged strenuous exercise could reduce delivery of oxygen and nutrients to the baby. Some studies in animals have indicated that overheating of the mother in the first trimester can cause birth defects and heighten the risk of neural tube defects. There are no reports that hyperthermia resulting from exercise causes malformations in humans; however, it makes sense to avoid exercise in the heat of the day, stay hydrated and avoid saunas or hot spas after your workout or, indeed, anytime during pregnancy. For all these reasons, swimming or exercise in water is often recommended. Not only does the buoyancy reduce the risk of injury to your joints, you are less likely to become overheated.

## Exercise considerations during pregnancy

As your pregnancy progresses, your ability to exercise can be affected:

- The increase in weight and change in body shape can make some types of exercise more difficult and uncomfortable.
- Your center of gravity changes as you begin to "show" during the second trimester, and this can affect your balance and increase the risk of falling.
- Your joints will loosen to prepare for birth and this can increase the risk of injury, particularly with high-impact exercise or excessive stretching.
- Your resting heart rate increases and your maximum heart rate decreases, so don't use heart-rate monitoring to determine the intensity of your exercise. Instead, it is better to monitor your perceived level of exertion.
- Blood pressure falls from the second trimester, which can cause you to feel light-headed or dizzy if you change positions quickly.

## BEST EXERCISE OPTIONS IN PREGNANCY

There are four considerations: type, intensity, duration and frequency of exercise.

Let's deal with type first. While yoga, Pilates and gentle stretching are excellent for pregnant women, additional aerobic exercise is recommended. Aerobic exercise means exercise of relatively low intensity but long duration, and it includes walking, hiking, jogging, running, dancing, aerobics, swimming, cycling and rowing. But from a clinical perspective, the best types of exercise during pregnancy are those without risk of falling, impact or overheating.

More vigorous sports should be decided on a case-by-case basis with your health-care professional, taking into consideration your history of participation in the sport. If you've jogged daily for most of your adult life, then it's probably fine to keep it up for as long as you're comfortable. If you've never skied before and want to attempt it at 30 weeks gestation, then think again.

But you should be careful not to overdo it. Use lighter weights and more repetitions, because heavy weights may overload joints already loosened by the increase in pregnancy hormones. Because of the relaxation of ligaments during pregnancy, only gentle stretching should be undertaken. Avoid walking lunges, because these may raise the risk of injury to connective tissue in the pelvis. In a trial of 160 pregnant women, those who performed light resistance exercise training three times per week for 35–40 minutes per session gained less weight during pregnancy than the control group.

Ideally, one or two of your exercise sessions each week should be devoted to muscle strengthening and stretching (one aerobic session can be replaced by a strength/stretch session). You should be using the larger muscle groups (for example, knee extensions, hamstring curls, bench press and bicep curls) with lighter weights. We recommend you halve the weight you normally lift and double the number of repetitions. If you normally do leg presses with 30 pounds for 8–12 reps, try 20 pounds for 15–20 reps. If you usually do chest presses with 20 pounds for 8–12 reps, try 10 pounds for 15–20 reps. You shouldn't lie flat on your back because this might cause the uterus to compress a major vein—instead, tilt the bench to an incline. If you are using free weights, be careful not to hit your belly. Inexpensive resistance bands are a good alternative to free weights, and you can use them at home rather than going to the gym.

## EXERCISE INTENSITY

Unless there are complications in your particular case, it is perfectly safe to engage in moderately intense exercise during pregnancy, and there are good reasons to perform vigorous exercise. Moderate intensity corresponds to a typical walking pace, or 3 on the Borg Scale of Perceived Exertion (see the box on the next page). You've increased your heart rate but you can still have a normal conversation with someone who is exercising with you. Engaging in vigorous exercise (5 on the Borg Scale) may be worthwhile because it has been linked to shorter duration of labor (which may not necessarily mean it's easier!). Obstetrician Dr. John Clapp found that previously active women who trained throughout all three trimesters experienced two hours less labor than the women who stopped exercising before the end of the first trimester.

The more vigorous the exercise, the less total time of exercise is required. For example, you could walk at a moderate pace (2.5 miles per hour, Borg 3) for 60 minutes on six days a week, or you could walk at a brisk pace (3.7 miles per hour, Borg 5) for 30 minutes on six days a week.

Whatever the intensity, you should always listen to your body. Due to increasing size and fatigue, very active women find that they naturally reduce the amount of exercise they do as their pregnancy progresses. By the third trimester, three 30-minute sessions of vigorous exercise per week is sufficient to maintain your cardiovascular fitness.

## Borgs Rating of Perceived Exertion Scale

| | |
|---|---|
| 0—Nothing at all | 6 |
| 1—Very light | 7—Very hard |
| 2—Fairly light | 8 |
| **3—Moderate** | 9 |
| 4—Somewhat hard | 10—Very, very hard |
| **5—Hard** | |

## Optimum amounts of exercise during pregnancy

Moderate exercise or moderate intensity resistance training = about 6 hours per week of walking at 2.5 miles per hour

OR

Vigorous (aerobic) exercise = about 3 hours per week of walking at 3.7 miles per hour

Note: 1 hour of vigorous exercise = 2 hours of moderate exercise

| SAMPLE WEEK OF SUGGESTED EXERCISE | |
|---|---|
| Monday | 30-minute walk in the early morning or late in the day |
| Tuesday | 60 minutes at the gym (20 minutes vigorous exercise, 40 minutes weights and stretches) |
| Wednesday | 30-minute walk in the early morning or late in the day |
| Thursday | 60 minutes at the gym (20 minutes vigorous exercise, 40 minutes weights and stretches) |
| Friday | 30-minute walk in the early morning or late in the day |
| Saturday | 60 minutes at the gym (20 minutes vigorous exercise, 40 minutes weights and stretches) |
| Sunday | 30-minute walk in the early morning or late in the day, or gardening |

## PRECAUTIONS

Exercise should be stopped if any abnormal symptoms occur, such as pain, contractions, vaginal bleeding, dizziness or unusual shortness of breath (see the box below). Exercise during pregnancy is not advised if you have a medical history of heart disease, severe hypertension (high blood pressure), premature labor (for example, incompetent cervix or ruptured membranes), multiple pregnancy (twins or more) or pre-eclampsia. Any illness or complication should be fully assessed and discussed with your doctor before commencing or continuing an exercise program.

### EXERCISES THAT REQUIRE CAUTION

During pregnancy, it's prudent to seek individualized medical advice for certain types of sports and activities. These include:

» Contact sports or activities that carry a risk of falling (such as snow skiing and horseback riding).

» Competition sports such as soccer, hockey and basketball. Consider the stage of pregnancy, the level of competition and your level of fitness.

» After about the fourth month of pregnancy, exercises that involve lying on your back—the weight of the baby can slow the return of blood to your heart. Try to modify these exercises by lying on the side.

» In the later stages of pregnancy, activities that involve jumping, frequent changes of direction and excessive stretching (such as gymnastics).

» Scuba diving should be avoided because the baby is at increased risk of decompression sickness.

### WARNING SIGNS

If you experience any of the following symptoms during or after exercise, you should stop and contact your doctor:

» High heart rate (which may cause heart palpitations)

» Chest pain

- » Dizziness or feeling faint
- » Headache
- » Uterine contractions
- » Vaginal bleeding
- » Amniotic fluid leakage
- » Nausea
- » Shortness of breath
- » Deep back pain or pelvic pain
- » A decrease or unusual change in your baby's movements
- » Sudden swelling of ankles, hands and face
- » Calf pain or swelling
- » Cramping in the lower abdomen
- » Walking difficulties.

To minimize the risk of harm, wear lightweight clothes and don't exercise outdoors in the heat of the day. If you are exercising indoors, keep the room well ventilated and drink plenty of water before, during and after your exercise session. Avoid exercise that carries a risk of falling (for example, outdoor walks on uneven terrain or outdoor cycling) or that is hard impact (such as boxing, running, jumping, skipping, contact sports and high-impact aerobics). Avoid any form of exercise at very high intensity, even if you were already doing this before you got pregnant. This is particularly important in the early stages of pregnancy to reduce the risk of miscarriage.

## THE "30 MINUTES A DAY" RULE

If you've been sedentary before pregnancy, you should follow a gradual progression up to 30 minutes a day on most, if not all, days of the week. Prolonged sessions in excess of 45 minutes of continuous exercise can be carried out as long as you are not at risk of overheating, of dehydration or food restriction. Be guided by how you feel and stop and rest when needed.

Exercise for 30 minutes a day—a lifelong goal.

The recommendation of 30 minutes a day is something to strive for not just during pregnancy but the rest of your life. It's something the whole family should aim for, and you're their role model. Getting your daily exercise should not be seen as selfish—it's like putting your own oxygen mask on before your child's: If you're fit, you're in a better position to look after them.

## ABDOMINAL EXERCISES AND PREGNANCY

The abdominal core and pelvic floor muscles act as a natural "corset" to protect your pelvis and spine. In other words, strong abdominal muscles will help protect you against back problems and pain. Conventional sit-ups or crunches are mostly ineffective during pregnancy and may make worse the condition known as "diastasis recti abdominis" (a painless splitting of the abdominal muscle at the midline).

Appropriate floor exercises are recommended during pregnancy to strengthen the muscles of the abdomen and lower back:

» Concentrate on drawing your belly button toward your spine.
» Breathe out while pulling in your belly.
» Hold the position and count to ten. Relax and breathe in.
» Repeat ten times, as many times a day as you are able.
» You can perform this exercise sitting, standing or on your hands and knees. (Avoid lying on your back from around the fourth month of pregnancy.)

### DON'T IGNORE THE PELVIC FLOOR

Your pelvic floor muscles are weakened during pregnancy and can be damaged during a vaginal delivery, so it's *extremely* important to condition them ("muscle them up") from the start of your pregnancy. These exercises (they are also known as Kegels) can be continued right through your pregnancy and restarted as soon as it feels comfortable after the birth of your baby. Indeed, Kegels can improve sexual function and increase the enjoyment of sex, a gentle form of exercise. A physiotherapist or midwife can show you how to do Kegels, or see the box on the next page for more details.

# Kegels (pelvic floor exercises)

**How to do pelvic floor exercises**

- Pull in the pelvic floor muscles and hold for a count of three.
- Release and relax for a count of three.
- Repeat ten times.
- Practice this three times every day, preferably once lying down, once while sitting and once while standing.

**Finding the pelvic floor muscles**

- It helps to imagine you are tightening your vagina around a tampon. The old tip of stopping and starting the flow of urine is no longer considered appropriate. Try *not* to contract your abs.

## POSTPARTUM EXERCISE

Many of the physiological changes of pregnancy persist for four to six weeks after delivery. In this period, called the postpartum period, try to resume the exercises you were doing in the third trimester soon after birth. Most women are perfectly capable of engaging in a gentle exercise routine within days of delivery, and there is some evidence that a return to physical activity helps reduce the chance of postpartum depression. A gradual return is advisable. Many women find that any form of bouncy exercise (such as jogging or aerobics) is rather uncomfortable, and it is reasonable to minimize this type of activity until the pelvic floor tightens up. Women who are breastfeeding might consider feeding their infants before exercising to avoid the discomfort of engorged breasts.

# Where to get help

- Your doctor
- An accredited exercise physiologist (AEP)
- Physical therapist—to find one near you, visit moveforward.com
- Personal trainer (ensure he or she is properly qualified and have experience in working with pregnant women)
- National Association for Continence (NAFC)—call 1-800-BLADDER or visit nafc.org.
- The Mayo Clinic—visit mayoclinic.com/health/pregnancy-and-exercise /PR00096 and mayoclinic.com/health/exercise-after-pregnancy/MY00477 for advice on exercise both during and after pregnancy.

## SUMMARY: EXERCISE IN PREGNANCY

Exercise during pregnancy offers many physical, emotional and often social benefits. Despite profound changes in your anatomy and physiology, exercise has minimal risks and confirmed benefits for most women. Engaging in sufficient moderate to vigorous exercise on most days of the week will optimize pregnancy weight gain and birth weight, and reduce the chances of developing gestational diabetes. While exercise during pregnancy is usually encouraged, you may feel it's not right for you. Talk to your doctor, exercise physiologist, physiotherapist or health-care professional to make sure your exercise routine won't cause harm to you or your unborn baby.

# Chapter 7

# Gestational diabetes: why such a big deal?

Gestational diabetes (strictly speaking, it's gestational diabetes mellitus, sometimes abbreviated to GDM) is the most common medical problem encountered during pregnancy. The name is derived from the combination of having a raised blood sugar level, as occurs in people with diabetes mellitus, and being pregnant (gestational). While "blood sugar" is the commonly used term, it is actually a measurement of glucose in a blood sample taken from a vein. In practice, the terms are used interchangeably.

## WHAT IS GESTATIONAL DIABETES?

Gestational diabetes is any degree of "glucose intolerance" diagnosed for the first time during pregnancy. Glucose tolerance refers to the body's ability to handle a large amount of glucose consumed in the fasting state. If blood glucose levels rise moderately and return to normal levels quickly, you are tolerant. If glucose levels rise to a very high level or remain high for some time, you are glucose intolerant. The definition of gestational diabetes refers to *any degree* rather than a specific glucose level, as diagnostic cut-offs vary in different countries. A small number of women may have unrecognized diabetes before pregnancy, or develop diabetes incidentally during their pregnancy. This is still referred to as gestational diabetes, but after delivery, their glucose levels will remain high, and the appropriate diagnosis (for example, type 1 or type 2 diabetes) can be made.

## WHAT DO GLUCOSE AND INSULIN DO?

Glucose circulates in the blood and is taken up by the cells and used for energy production. Excess glucose can also be converted and stored as fat. The glucose circulating in the blood comes from what the body makes and also from what we eat. Most of the carbohydrates in foods, whether in the form of starch or sugar, are digested and broken down to glucose for absorption. Thus a measurement of the glucose level in the blood reflects both what the body is making and what is being absorbed after eating.

Insulin is a hormone produced in special cells called "beta" cells, found in the pancreas. The pancreas sits behind the stomach and is responsible for producing the enzymes and juices needed for digestion. Insulin is secreted into the blood and assists the passage of glucose from the blood to the cells. After we eat, the pancreas detects the rapid rise in glucose and, under normal circumstances, releases an amount of insulin appropriate to the size of the glucose load. If some resistance is detected, the beta cells simply secrete more insulin. As the glucose level in the blood falls, the amount of insulin being released also gradually falls.

## WHAT ARE THE DIFFERENT TYPES OF DIABETES?

Type 1 diabetes, previously known as juvenile-onset diabetes or insulin-dependent diabetes mellitus (IDDM), is the type of diabetes that is commonly found in younger people, usually has a sudden onset and is due to an absolute deficiency of insulin—the insulin-secreting cells in the pancreas have been largely destroyed and no insulin is produced. All people with type 1 diabetes need insulin injections.

Type 2 diabetes, previously known as maturity-onset diabetes or non-insulin-dependent diabetes (NIDDM) is the type of diabetes that is commonly found in older people, although it is increasingly being diagnosed in younger adults and even children. It usually comes on gradually (or is found accidentally, for example on routine blood tests) and is due to worsening resistance to the actions of insulin. For a variety of reasons, including genetic background, excess body fat, diet and lifestyle, the available insulin is not sufficient to overcome the resistance. Often people with this problem will have raised levels of insulin—the insulin is simply not producing the desired effect. This can be controlled by changes to diet or using tablets. Over the course of time, however, the hard-working insulin-secreting beta cells become exhausted and can no longer produce sufficient insulin to control blood glucose levels. A state of relative or absolute insulin deficiency develops, and insulin injections may be needed.

Gestational diabetes is closely related to type 2 diabetes, and a significant proportion of women with gestational diabetes will go on to develop type 2 diabetes later in life. In this case, the metabolic stress of pregnancy has temporarily unmasked a susceptibility that will be exposed again later in life.

## HISTORICAL PERSPECTIVE

A little history helps us understand how the treatment of gestational diabetes has evolved over time. A century ago, the discovery of insulin meant both males and females with type 1 diabetes no longer died at a young age, but females still had a very poor outlook when it came to pregnancy. Not only were they less likely to become pregnant, they also had a higher rate of miscarriage and other pregnancy complications. A higher rate of adverse pregnancy outcomes was also observed in women who were normal during the pregnancy but found later to have developed diabetes (usually type 2). These women, in fact, probably had minor degrees of glucose abnormalities during the pregnancy that went unrecognized. It has become recognized that the potentially harmful effects of a raised glucose level during pregnancy ranged from glucose levels that were undoubtedly high to glucose levels that were only slightly elevated. There is, in fact, a continuum of risk, and even minor elevations of maternal glucose can be associated with some degree of measurable risk.

Concerns about gestational diabetes have therefore changed markedly over the past fifty years. Initially, glucose testing in pregnancy was used to identify a mother at higher risk of developing type 2 diabetes. In the 1990s, however, when the risk of a moderately high glucose level became clear, consideration of testing of all women at the beginning of the third trimester was recommended in the United States and many other countries. In the past ten years, the concept known as "intrauterine programming" has risen to prominence. Studies showed that the mother's glucose level and diet, in general, had a profound influence on the metabolism and programming of a baby in the womb. In other words, what you eat during pregnancy can influence your baby's birth weight, body fat, food preferences and the development of diseases in later life (as we discussed earlier, in Chapters 3 and 4).

It's now clear that our chances of developing diabetes later in life are dependent not only on our genetic background, diet and lifestyle, but also on the circumstances under which we were conceived and our experiences in utero. Research suggests that approximately half of the number of cases of diabetes in later life may be due to higher glucose levels during pregnancy. If this is the case, then this is also potentially reversible and controllable.

## EPIGENETICS

Epigenetics refers to the study of changes in genes and gene expression caused by mechanisms *other than* mutations. It used to be thought that we were all born with a unique DNA fingerprint that was set for life at the time of conception and, in time, passed onto our children. If we noticed an overweight child with two slim parents, we blamed the child's lifestyle, perhaps a poor diet and lack of exercise, not their genes.

But we now know that the environment, particularly experienced in utero, can change the way our genes are expressed. We also know that we are born with far more genes than we can ever use; which ones we use and how they are used are influenced by a large number of factors, including lifestyle changes within one generation. This can then be passed on because of specific "marks" left on the genes.

Think of a builder asked to build a house and given more material than required. Now the function of houses over hundreds of years has not changed, but the style, color and design has. Thus a builder will be able to use the different arrangements of materials to make houses that are all in some way different but still retain the fundamentals.

In the same way, dietary factors during pregnancy, both good and bad, can leave marks on the DNA of unborn children. Dietary influences may not alter the final height or the color of their eyes, but it can alter the risks of metabolic problems, such as obesity and diabetes, in later life.

## INTRAUTERINE PROGRAMMING

As we've seen, what you eat during pregnancy will affect your baby. The glucose in your blood crosses the placenta and is the major source of energy for the baby. But your insulin does not. Thus, from a very early age, the baby has to make its own insulin, and the amount being produced will depend on your glucose levels. If your glucose levels are raised, then the baby takes what it needs to develop normally—and then takes the extra glucose and makes fat.

Not only does your glucose cross the placenta and influence what happens to the developing baby, but probably everything you eat can have an influence. Studies in animals can provide data that would be impossible to obtain in humans. In one study, pregnant rats were fed either a boring rat chow or a junk-food diet (high in saturated fats and sugars) throughout their pregnancy. At birth, the pups were given to substitute mothers. When later challenged with various food choices, the pups whose mothers had consumed the poor diet selectively consumed more of the junk foods.

## WHY IS GESTATIONAL DIABETES IMPORTANT?

A diagnosis of gestational diabetes is important for many reasons. First, it identifies women who may be at risk for developing type 2 diabetes later in life. The forewarning means they can make diet and lifestyle changes, for themselves and their family, to help reduce their chances. Some women, during and after pregnancy, may also be prescribed metformin, a drug that reduces insulin resistance and may prevent or delay the development of diabetes.

Second, women with gestational diabetes are more likely to have a large baby. While women without diabetes can also have big babies, the reasons are different and often genetically determined (for example, both the mother and father are tall). Women with gestational diabetes have bigger babies because high amounts of glucose are converted and stored as fat around the baby's abdomen. The increased size of the baby's abdomen can be detected and measured on ultrasound.

A mother with a large baby, whatever the cause, is more likely to have a complicated delivery, with injury to both the baby and the mother. There is an increased rate of medical intervention (for example, forceps delivery) and higher rates of both elective and emergency Caesarean section. In many instances, the detection of a large baby will mean an earlier delivery is scheduled with induction of labor.

Women with gestational diabetes are also at increased risk of having a baby with a *low* glucose level after delivery. This is because of the sudden withdrawal of the mother's high glucose supply and the baby's relatively high insulin level. For this reason, together with additional concerns, the baby may need to be admitted to a neonatal intensive care unit. These complications are directly related to the higher glucose levels in the mother. The good news is that they are highly unlikely if the diabetes is properly treated and glucose levels are normal.

Finally, gestational diabetes is now a concern because of what we now know of programming in the womb and the potential for your baby to be more at risk of developing diseases in later life. What you eat during pregnancy affects the way the baby develops and the food choices that your baby will make later in life. It is not just your blood glucose levels that are important but all aspects of your diet. However, because carbohydrates are responsible for the rise and fall in your glucose levels after eating, carbohydrate foods are given special attention. Foods with a low glycemic index will lead to a smaller rise and fall in the glucose levels, and these gradual changes are passed through the placenta to the baby. Foods with a high glycemic index will cause a rapid rise in your blood glucose, and this glucose spike is passed through to the baby. For complex reasons related to the circulation of the amniotic fluid, this spike can have a sustained effect.

## ARE YOU AT RISK OF GESTATIONAL DIABETES?

There are many different risk factors that predict the risk of developing diabetes during pregnancy. One or more of these may be operating in different women.

# RISK FACTORS THAT CANNOT BE AVOIDED

1.  If there is a family history of type 2 diabetes, then there is likely to be a genetically determined tendency to develop the problem. The average age of diagnosis of type 2 diabetes has been falling. A negative family history is not necessarily reassuring as some women in their pregnancy may not yet have a first-degree relation who is old enough to have developed or been diagnosed with diabetes.

2.  Gestational diabetes is more common in women who come from an ethnic background with a higher overall rate of diabetes or an earlier age of onset. This includes, but is not confined to African Americans, Hispanic/Latino Americans, American Indians, Asian Americans and Pacific Islander Americans.

3.  Increasing age of mothers. With women now delaying their families often until their thirties, they are much further advanced toward the time when they potentially may develop type 2 diabetes in the future. Therefore, under the stress of pregnancy, this problem can be unmasked.

4.  A previous adverse obstetric history. There is an increased risk of developing gestational diabetes in women who have had previous miscarriages, large babies and adverse pregnancy outcomes. This group is becoming less and less common as routine testing for gestational diabetes becomes more established.

5.  A previous history of gestational diabetes. Women who have had gestational diabetes in one pregnancy are much more likely to develop this again in subsequent pregnancies. However, this is by no means inevitable and there is generally about a 50 percent recurrence rate. This rate can be reduced by careful attention to diet between the pregnancies, particularly with respect to reducing the intake of saturated fat.

6.  Women with PCOS have a much higher risk of developing gestational diabetes. The underlying problem in PCOS is insulin resistance, the same problem that occurs in type 2 diabetes, and these women are also at higher risk of developing type 2 diabetes later in life.

## RISK FACTORS THAT CAN BE REVERSED OR AVOIDED

1.  Women who are overweight are much more likely to develop gestational diabetes. The more overweight they are, the higher the probability. Independent of any abnormality with their blood sugar level, women who are overweight are also much more likely to have large babies. Research shows that serious attention to diet and exercise can reduce your chances of developing gestational diabetes and/or delivering a large baby.
2.  A poor diet, both before and during pregnancy. Many women report unusual food cravings during early pregnancy, sometimes for foods that are less than optimal (for example, chips). While one food doesn't make or break a good diet, a reasonable question is whether a consistently poor diet can cause gestational diabetes. We know from animal research that the answer is yes, but similar experiments would be unethical in humans. We do know that women diagnosed with gestational diabetes who follow dietary advice are able to significantly lower their blood sugar levels. Thus, it is likely that a less-than-healthy diet during pregnancy may unmask a tendency toward gestational diabetes.
3.  Women who exercise regularly are less likely to develop gestational diabetes. In fact, studies have shown that women who are most active before pregnancy have less than half the risk of developing gestational diabetes compared to those who are least active, and those with the highest activity levels in early pregnancy reduce their risk of gestational diabetes by around 25 percent compared to those who are inactive. Studies have also shown that pregnant women can use exercise to lower elevated glucose levels. If gestational diabetes does eventuate, then exercise will be an important part of your management plan. (See Chapter 6 for details on what to do and precautions.)

## SHOULD ALL WOMEN BE TESTED OR JUST THOSE WITH RISK FACTORS?

All women should be tested for gestational diabetes in every pregnancy. Women with risk factors are more likely to have gestational diabetes, but women with no risk factors at all can also have this problem.

## DIAGNOSIS

The diagnosis of gestational diabetes is made by measuring the glucose level in a blood sample taken from a vein (venous glucose). The finger-prick glucose meters, while useful for monitoring, are not accurate enough for diagnostic purposes. The diagnosis of gestational diabetes can be made at any time during pregnancy. A significantly raised result (such as a fasting glucose greater than or equal to 126 mg/dl or a random glucose greater than or equal to 200 mg/dl) is likely to represent preexisting diabetes in someone who is also pregnant. This will be determined by formal testing after the baby has been delivered.

Women who are considered to be at high risk for gestational diabetes (for example, women who have developed it in a previous pregnancy) are usually tested in the first trimester. Women not known to have either diabetes or gestational diabetes require testing at around 24–28 weeks gestation. There are two methods currently available for this.

1.  The older method, which is currently endorsed by the American College of Obstetricians and Gynecologists, requires all women to be considered for testing at this time. Some women may have a preliminary glucose challenge test (GCT), which requires 50 grams of glucose in the non-fasting state (that is, at any time), and a three-hour GTT on a different day only if the one-hour sample of the GCT is 140 mg/dl or higher. The definitive test requires an oral glucose tolerance test after an overnight fast with a 100-gram glucose load and four blood tests. It is the most commonly used GTT, and is considered abnormal if values of glucose are higher than normal in two or more of the blood tests. Thus, for many women testing becomes a two-stage procedure.

The following values are considered abnormal during this GTT:

| INTERVAL | ABNORMAL READING |
| --- | --- |
| Fasting | 95 mg/dl or higher |
| One hour | 180 mg/dl or higher |
| Two hours | 155 mg/dl or higher |
| Three hours | 140 mg/dl or higher |

2. The newer method, endorsed by the American Diabetes Association, is much simpler. All women are recommended to be tested, because a decision about who to test based on risk factors will certainly miss some women with gestational diabetes. For the same reason, the GCT is no longer recommended. The dose of glucose used in the new method (75 grams) is lower than that used in the old method, and the complete test lasts only two hours and requires just three blood samples. A diagnosis of gestational diabetes is made if one of the results is raised.

The following values are considered abnormal during this GTT:

| INTERVAL | ABNORMAL READING |
| --- | --- |
| Fasting | 92 mg/dl or higher |
| One hour | 180 mg/dl or higher |
| Two hours | 153 mg/dl or higher |

When preparing for a GTT, it is common to ask women to have a high carbohydrate intake for the three days before the test. For any person eating a reasonable amount of carbohydrates, this is unnecessary but is still done by some laboratories, mainly for historical reasons. The glucose levels used to define the results of the GTT are different in different parts of the world. In the United States, the preferred GTT for testing is still being debated.

## THE RISKS IN OLDER MOTHERS

For a variety of reasons, the average age in pregnancy has been gradually increasing over the last fifty years. Increasing age is a major risk factor for the development of gestational diabetes because insulin resistance worsens as we age, irrespective of gender. Thus women who are contemplating a pregnancy in their late thirties and even forties need to be particularly aware. Early testing in pregnancy can be a distinct advantage and reveal any abnormality that may be present.

## WHAT SHOULD THE TARGET GLUCOSE LEVELS BE?

Like the diagnostic criteria, the target levels are in a state of transition and no firm recommendations have been made. However, it would be logical to aim for a fasting glucose level less than the level of whichever diagnostic test was used. Whether to test one or two hours after meals and what levels should be aimed for is a decision your obstetric-care provider can make with you.

# DIETARY MANAGEMENT OF GESTATIONAL DIABETES

As we've described in other sections of this book, all women with gestational diabetes should receive advice about diet and lifestyle. The cornerstone of managing gestational diabetes is modifying your diet. In fact, for the majority of women diagnosed with gestational diabetes, dietary management is the *only* treatment that is necessary. A carbohydrate-controlled diet, evenly distributed throughout the day and with a predominance of low GI food choices, is the ideal. Insulin or other medications will only be added if dietary changes and moderate physical activity are unable to keep your blood glucose levels in the target range.

The eating guidelines that are given in Part 4 are suitable for all women who are pregnant, with or without gestational diabetes. The only difference if you have gestational diabetes is the need to be more careful with the quantities of food you eat, particularly of carbohydrate-containing foods. As discussed in Chapter 5, carbohydrates are the dietary component that immediately affects your blood glucose levels.

If you consume carbohydrates that are quickly digested and absorbed (those with a high GI) or eat a large amount of carbohydrates in one sitting, regardless of GI, your blood glucose levels may rise too high. The key to managing your blood glucose levels is to have a fairly consistent intake of carbohydrates spread over three meals and snacks and to choose mostly low GI varieties.

> Maintain a consistent intake of low GI carbohydrates spread over three meals and snacks.

In earlier chapters, we explained the numerous benefits of choosing low GI carbohydrates when you are pregnant, and this is particularly important when you have gestational diabetes. High GI carbohydrates can lead to a sudden, high peak in your blood sugar levels, giving a "pulse" of glucose to your baby, causing him or her to secrete more insulin. Over time, the high insulin level increases your baby's rate of growth, with the potential to cause high birth weight, excess body fat and more complicated deliveries.

The appropriate amount of carbohydrates for you depends on several factors, including your weight, how active you are and your rate of weight gain. If at all possible, we recommend seeing a dietitian, who'll be able to give you specific advice on your individual needs. However, a general guide is to include two to three servings of carbohydrate-containing foods at meals and one serving between meals. One serving or portion (also called an "exchange") is considered the amount of a particular food that provides about 15 grams of carbohydrates. (The 15 grams is not the weight of the food, but the amount of carbohydrates it contains when eaten.) Some examples and equivalent exchanges are shown below.

| BREADS AND CRACKERS | | FRUITS | |
|---|---|---|---|
| Bread | 1 slice | Apple | 1 medium |
| Dinner roll | ½ large or 1 small | Banana | 1 small |
| Ryvita® or Kavli crispbreads | 2 | Kiwi | 2 |
| | | Mandarin | 2 medium |
| Stoned Wheat Thins | 10 | Orange | 1 medium |
| **RICE AND PASTA** | | Peach | 1 large |
| Basmati rice | cooked ⅓ cup | Pear | 1 medium |
| Pasta | cooked ½ cup | Dried apricots | 5 |
| Noodles | cooked ½ cup | **DAIRY PRODUCTS** | |
| **BREAKFAST CEREALS** | | Milk | 8 ounces |
| All-Bran® | ½ cup | Plain yogurt | 6 ounces |
| Soy Crunch Multi-Grain Cereal | ¾ cup | Ice cream | 2 scoops |
| Rolled oats | ¼ cup raw | | |
| **STARCHY VEGETABLES** | | | |
| Sweet potato (any kind) | ½ cup | | |
| Corn | 1 medium cob | | |
| Baked beans | ½ cup | | |
| Lentils | ½ cup | | |

In addition to carbohydrate foods, you can eat as many non-starchy vegetables and salads as you like (for example, green vegetables, bell peppers, carrots, tomatoes and salad greens), and moderate amounts of lean protein such as lean meat, chicken, fish, eggs and tofu.

Many women with gestational diabetes are advised to have two carbohydrate portions at breakfast, such as two slices of low GI whole grain bread. To this, you could add one poached egg (a protein source) and grilled tomatoes and mushrooms (neither of which contain significant amounts of carbohydrates). The same applies to the evening meal. You could choose a cup of noodles (your two carbohydrate portions) with a selection of stir-fry vegetables, and some chicken breast or tofu to complete the meal.

Women diagnosed with gestational diabetes are also recommended to undertake home glucose monitoring using a finger-prick device. This experience teaches you how different foods are digested and absorbed in your body. You'll see for yourself that some foods send your blood glucose levels up too high, while others don't, and are, therefore, better choices. In this respect, having gestational diabetes is a valuable learning opportunity for the rest of your life. By adopting a healthy low GI diet in the long term, you'll be able to reduce your risk of developing type 2 diabetes, and guide your whole family toward better food choices.

Following a low GI diet can help to keep blood glucose levels on target and reduce the chances you will need insulin. In a study carried out among women with a diagnosis of gestational diabetes in Wollongong, Australia, we found that those who were instructed to follow a low GI diet were half as likely to require insulin treatment as those given directions to follow a conventional healthy diet.

## TARGET GLUCOSE LEVELS

Target glucose levels for women with gestational diabetes vary from one diabetes center to another.

As a general guideline:

» First thing in the morning: less than 95 mg/dl
» One-hour post-meal glucose level: less than 140 mg/dl
» Two-hour post-meal glucose level: less than 120 mg/dl

Nonetheless, it is important that you don't overly restrict your diet for the sake of your blood glucose levels. Your baby's growth is still dependent on your eating sufficient amounts of healthy food. If your blood glucose levels are consistently elevated despite a healthy low GI diet and appropriate physical activity, then it is time to start insulin or medication. This is not a failure on your part, but simply a reflection that your beta cells are not coping with the higher demand for insulin that accompanies every pregnancy, gestational diabetes or not.

Many women with gestational diabetes find that blood glucose levels are most likely to be high after breakfast. This is the one meal where carbohydrate foods dominate (think cereal and toast), so choosing low GI options to start the day is more critical. For some women mornings are also a time of rushing and stress. Any stress will release stress hormones and these have an anti-insulin action—if your insulin action is already compromised, then this will increase your glucose levels. Reducing the pressures at this time by getting up ten to fifteen minutes earlier and taking time to sit and eat a relaxing breakfast may help. The evening meal can also be a problem, particularly if you are accustomed to having large servings of pasta or rice. It is fine to include these foods, but they need to be in measured amounts and combined with plenty of vegetables or salad and some protein.

Spreading your food out over the day will help to manage your blood glucose levels by avoiding large quantities of food at one time. Toward the end of pregnancy, there may be a tendency to go to bed earlier and sleep longer. This may mean that your meals all get pushed into a relatively short period during the day and there is a long gap overnight. It is better if you can avoid this, even if it means an early start and having a nap or rest later in the day, if possible. As a general rule, the evening meal should be ten hours or more after breakfast.

Be wary of products marketed as "suitable for diabetics," "no added sugar" or "low-carb." Many of them are high in calories and saturated fat and are not a good choice. Some contain low-digestible carbohydrates that can cause digestive symptoms, such as gas, bloating and diarrhea. Similarly, be careful with foods marketed as "low-fat," some of which may be higher in total or high GI carbohydrates.

If you follow these eating guidelines, in combination with moderate exercise, there is a good chance you can manage your blood glucose levels without the need for insulin or medication, and you will reduce any risks to your baby of being exposed to excess glucose.

## The "6 out of 7" rule

If you think about the 21 major meals each week, then you are probably responsible for at least 18 of them (seven breakfasts, five lunches, six evening meals or similar combination). Thus the "6 out of 7" rule implies that when you're in charge, take charge. It's your responsibility to choose a healthy meal at these times. On the other occasions, when you're not in charge, sit back, relax and enjoy.

## TREATING GESTATIONAL DIABETES

A low GI diet will reduce your chances of starting additional therapy, such as insulin. Ask your doctor if you can have a trial of diet before other treatments are contemplated. If target glucose levels are not being met on your diet, then treatment with either insulin or different sorts of pills can be considered.

At this stage of our knowledge, insulin is the preferred treatment and the default option if pills don't appear to be working. If gestational diabetes is diagnosed early in pregnancy, a trial of pills can be undertaken, but if target glucose levels are not reached by 30 weeks gestation, then insulin should be started.

## TREATMENT WITH INSULIN

Gestational diabetes develops because of increasing resistance to the normal actions of insulin, plus the inability to make enough insulin to meet the higher demand. Adding external insulin by way of injections can help the body overcome the problem. Insulin can only be given by injections (under the skin). For obvious reasons, this is not an attractive option for the majority of women. However, the reality is that once started, they find insulin injections about the same degree or less of an inconvenience as doing finger-prick blood glucose testing (which they are obliged to do regardless).

Modern insulins are available in the usual vials or as a disposable pen device that can be easily and safely carried around. The type of insulin and frequency will depend upon the pattern of glucose levels. It is quite common to use insulin twice daily (with breakfast and with the evening meal) using a formulation that is premixed, that is, containing both quick and long-acting varieties.

The insulin is usually injected with a short needle into the fat just underneath the skin of your stomach. The needles are never, ever long enough to reach anywhere near the baby. Insulin needs to be combined with diet changes, and the dose will be gradually adjusted to keep glucose levels within the target range. Provided correct attention is paid to the carbohydrate portions, there is only a very low risk of developing a low-sugar reaction (hypoglycemia).

## TREATMENT WITH PILLS

Recent research indicates that certain types of pills for diabetes are both safe and effective to use during pregnancy.

**Metformin** is a well-known oral medication that has been prescribed for people with diabetes for the past fifty years. It has been used in women with gestational diabetes for more than thirty years. Metformin acts by making the liver produce less glucose, and also by making the body more sensitive to insulin. An extended-release preparation is available that can be taken just once a day. The only significant side effects of taking metformin are tummy upsets with nausea, wind and, occasionally, diarrhea. These side effects are often dose-related and a smaller dose may not cause any symptoms at all. A large body of research indicates that there are no adverse pregnancy outcomes associated with its use. Continuing follow-up studies in the children of women who were prescribed metformin during pregnancy demonstrate no cause for concern.

**Glyburide** is a well-established oral medication that works by stimulating the beta cells in the pancreas to produce more insulin. Research has shown that it does not cross the placenta (or does so in very small amounts) and does not result in any adverse pregnancy outcomes. Your physician may prescribe a small dose and gradually increase it depending upon the response. Glyburide lasts a long time in the body and sometimes can lead to low glucose reactions.

## HOW AND WHEN DO I MONITOR MY GLUCOSE LEVELS?

If you are diagnosed with gestational diabetes, you will be asked to check your blood sugar levels on a regular basis. There are a variety of small portable devices (home glucose monitors) that can measure glucose levels with blood obtained by a finger-prick sample. While these are not accurate enough for diagnosis, they are generally accurate enough for monitoring.

Naturally, the intensity of monitoring is a compromise between, on one hand, the need for information and, on the other hand, the inconvenience and mild discomfort. There are many different advice options as to when glucose monitoring should be done. If the diet is consistent, then there is no need to test every day. The results after meals are most important, because these reflect not only the magnitude of glucose levels before a meal but the increase that has been caused by the carbohydrates in the diet. In pregnancy, glucose levels in the blood reach their peak at about one hour after the end of a meal (in the nonpregnant state, the peak occurs at 30 minutes). The higher the one-hour post-meal glucose level, the higher the accumulation of excess abdominal fat in the baby. Many women actually prefer to test at the one-hour mark, but testing at other times can also be used as convenient with different target glucose levels (as described below).

The most common advice is to test and record results first thing in the morning (fasting, before anything to eat) and either one or two hours after starting each of the three major meals.

## LABOR AND DELIVERY

If you are on pills or insulin, then you may need special consideration at the time of delivery. Your medications are being used to help control the growth of your baby rather than treating your diabetes directly. This is in contrast to a woman who has type 1 or type 2 diabetes prior to pregnancy. Therefore, at the onset of labor, whether spontaneous or induced, your medications can be safely suspended and no special precautions will be necessary.

Ideally, glyburide should be suspended 24 hours before delivery and metformin at least 12 hours before delivery. Under normal circumstances there is no need to have any insulin injections after labor has commenced.

Sometimes women who are on a high total daily dose of insulin may need to have an approximate half dose on the evening before induction or a Caesarean section. It would be unusual to require any insulin or insulin infusions during labor and delivery.

After your baby is safely delivered, no routine treatment is required, although we recommend that you continue finger-pricking for a day or so to make sure that glucose levels have returned to normal.

## HOW CAN I REDUCE MY RISK FOR NEXT TIME?

While having had gestational diabetes once is a major risk factor for having gestational diabetes in subsequent pregnancies, it's by no means definite. The rate of recurrence varies, but is usually around 50 percent. In other words, you have roughly a one in two chance of having gestational diabetes in the next pregnancy. Many women make dietary and lifestyle changes that improve insulin action and reduce their risk the second time around. Some studies suggest that women who avoid gestational diabetes the second time have significantly reduced their intake of fat between the pregnancies. Lower fat intake, especially of saturated fats, makes the body more sensitive to the available insulin—in other words, it reduces insulin resistance.

There are other strategies that can improve the odds of not developing diabetes again. If you are overweight, then gradual weight reduction between the pregnancies will be extremely helpful. If you have not been doing regular exercise, then starting and maintaining a program will not only help control your weight, but also improve insulin sensitivity.

## WHAT DIET SHOULD I FOLLOW AFTER PREGNANCY?

The healthy low GI diet that we recommend during pregnancy is exactly the same diet that you should follow in the future. This maximizes satiety and optimizes insulin sensitivity. There's no longer the same need to be consistent from meal to meal or day to day in the amount of carbohydrates (although we still advise women to include some low GI carbs in every meal). In Part 4 we show you how easy it is to follow and enjoy a healthy low GI diet.

# FREQUENTLY ASKED QUESTIONS

**"Will my baby be born with diabetes?"**

There is no increased risk of any baby being born with diabetes because their mother has gestational diabetes. However, a family history of diabetes is one of the known risk factors for developing diabetes at some later stage in life. If blood glucose levels are not properly managed during pregnancy (as we discussed earlier in this chapter), your child will have an additional risk factor for developing type 2 diabetes.

**"Will I be able to breastfeed?"**

Having gestational diabetes has no bearing at all on the decision to breastfeed (or not). Breastfeeding has multiple benefits for your baby that apply equally to mothers with and without diabetes (see Chapter 8). Breastfeeding can also have distinct positive advantages for you. Evidence is mounting that your chances of developing gestational diabetes again in a subsequent pregnancy, or type 2 diabetes later in life, are reduced if you breastfeed. Full breastfeeding until your baby is at least four to six months of age is recommended.

**"Why is my fasting glucose level high when I have not eaten anything overnight?"**

Much of the glucose in the blood comes from what you eat. However, the body is also constantly making glucose, especially overnight. Sometimes the fasting glucose level in the morning is the highest level for the whole day. This does not mean you are doing anything wrong but simply an indication that your liver is particularly resistant to the action of insulin. Clinical experience suggests that a low GI snack, such as a glass of milk, some yogurt, fruit or a slice of whole grain toast, before going to bed may sometimes solve the problem.

**"What causes my glucose to be elevated when I have done nothing different?"**

Your glucose level can be elevated if you are under stress of any sort. The stress hormone, cortisol, spikes whenever there is a physical or mental challenge. Cortisol ensures that the liver makes more glucose to meet the demand and makes the available insulin less efficient. A demanding job, rushing about, family issues or an unrelated illness such as a cold are all stressors. Just getting children off to school can be a challenge. If at all possible, it is better to try and plan ways to reduce this— even if it means getting out of bed a little earlier. Other factors, including infection and poor sleep, may also increase glucose levels.

**"When I checked my glucose level, it was very high, and then five minutes later it was normal. Why is this?"**

This usually happens because of some contaminating substance on the finger. A common example might be fruit or fruit juice. If it is not possible to wash your fingers every time before testing, then discard the first drop of blood (which will have effectively washed the skin) and test the second drop.

## SUMMARY: GESTATIONAL DIABETES

Gestational diabetes is now a common problem with serious implications. Every woman should be tested for diabetes in pregnancy. Treatment with diet, pills or insulin is very effective. The most important reasons for testing and treating are to reduce the risks associated with having a large baby and the effects of programming on your baby's future health.

Mothers-to-be with a diagnosis of gestational diabetes should:

1. Eat small regular meals and snacks spread over the day.
2. Try to maintain a similar intake of carbohydrate foods from day to day (a dietitian can give you advice on the right amount of carbohydrates for you).
3. Aim to choose mostly low glycemic index foods.
4. Combine your carbohydrates with plenty of vegetables and salads, lean protein and healthy fats at each meal.
5. Let home glucose monitoring guide your food choices, but remember not to starve for the sake of your blood sugars.

# SUMMARY
## 13 steps to growing a healthy baby

*Maintaining healthy lifestyle habits and taking steps to avoid harm throughout your pregnancy will ensure that your baby has the best possible start in life. Remember these important factors while you are pregnant:*

1.  If you smoke, stop.
2.  Avoid alcohol.
3.  Restrict caffeine intake.
4.  Eat a nutrient-dense diet—remember you need nutrition for two but not calories for two.
5.  Practice good food hygiene and avoid high-risk foods (those which may be contaminated with *Listeria, Salmonella* or *Toxoplasmosis*), liver and fish high in mercury.
6.  Exercise regularly but stick to moderate intensity, low-impact exercises.
7.  Aim for a healthy weight gain while avoiding gaining excess weight.
8.  Take folate and iodine supplements or a prenatal vitamin, but check with your doctor first if you have thyroid problems.
9.  If you don't eat fish or other sources of omega-3, consider taking a fish oil supplement or algal DHA supplement (suitable for vegetarians and vegans).
10. Try to get some sun exposure (according to safe exposure guidelines depending on where you live) and have your vitamin D levels checked—if they are low you will need a supplement.
11. Don't take any medications (prescription or nonprescription) or supplements without first checking that they are safe during pregnancy.
12. Limit exposure to harmful chemicals, including some household cleaning agents.
13. Be tested for gestational diabetes at around 26–28 weeks of pregnancy, or earlier if you are at higher risk. If you are found to have gestational diabetes, ensure you keep your blood glucose levels in the target range.

# Beyond Due-Day—you and your new baby

*Paying attention to your diet doesn't end with the delivery of your baby. Indeed, if you breastfeed, the demand for food energy and micronutrients increases substantially. Once lactation finishes, it's still your duty to be a good role model for your growing child. In Part 3, we describe how your nutritional needs change after birth, the benefits of breastfeeding for both you and your baby, the most common problems (is he or she getting enough milk?) and finally, the optimal weaning foods for baby. Because it's relatively common, we also discuss the warning signs of postpartum depression.*

# Chapter 8

# Lactation and looking after yourself

The demands of looking after a newborn baby can mean little time for you. But now is the time when looking after yourself is even more important, to ensure you are able to cope with your new role and the challenges it brings. In this chapter, we discuss the benefits of breastfeeding for both you and your baby, and we also reassure those mothers who, for a variety of reasons, choose formula feeding. We answer the most frequently asked questions, such as "Is my baby getting enough milk?" and "Do I need supplements while breastfeeding?," as well as common concerns such as "How do I get my figure back?" and "When can I restart my exercise routine?" Finally, we cover one of the more common experiences beyond delivery: postpartum depression.

## EATING WELL POST-PREGNANCY

Eating well, and regularly, can be more of a challenge once baby arrives, as finding the time to eat between feeding, changing, bathing and rocking a new infant isn't easy. Moreover, if you are on maternity leave, some members of the family may be under the false impression you have plenty of time on your hands to do the housework, shopping, meal preparation, care for other children *and* look after the new addition to the family.

If ever there was a time when you could enjoy more food, then this is it! Most women don't consume more energy during pregnancy, but they certainly do during lactation. If you plan to fully breastfeed (and this is recommended whenever possible), then every calorie that your baby requires for the first four to six months of life comes directly from you. Apart from vitamin D, your breasts provide all the building blocks of proteins, fats, carbohydrates and other vital factors that are needed for growth. And in those first precious few months, your infant is growing at the fastest rate that it *ever* will, even faster than it will in adolescence.

About three quarters of American women choose to breastfeed their babies in the first weeks of life. Unfortunately, many women give it up far too early. There are good reasons you should continue as long as possible, for your benefit as much as your baby's.

In more ways than one, your mammary glands are amazing organs. They will grow in size and weight throughout pregnancy as well as lactation. At peak lactation, they will be making about 34 ounces of milk a day. If you've been small-breasted all your life, then you might enjoy the extra "assets." During pregnancy, the mammary glands are growing rapidly under the influence of pregnancy hormones, particularly estrogen, progesterone and prolactin. High levels of estrogen and progesterone during pregnancy inhibit milk production, but following delivery of your baby and placenta, levels fall sharply, and prolactin comes into its own. Breast milk begins to flow.

Suckling itself induces a series of hormonal responses. When your baby's lips touch your nipple, prolactin is secreted by a gland in the brain, inducing the release of another hormone called oxytocin, which causes a reflex action known as the "let down" reflex (like a "knee jerk" reaction). Milk flows from the stores inside your breasts into the milk ducts that converge at the nipple. It will continue to flow as long as your baby suckles. Each time you nurse your infant, nerve impulses from the nipples to the hypothalamus (the command center) in your brain increase prolactin release by as much as tenfold. This lasts for about one hour each time you feed. Oxytocin secretion increases, too, but only momentarily.

Your body maintains lactation for as long as you and your baby wish. It's under fine feedback control, so that you synthesize only the milk that your baby withdraws. If you feed frequently and allow your baby to suckle for as long as they like, you'll always make sufficient milk for their needs. There is an art to breastfeeding, an art that most new moms need to learn from an experienced person, for example, their own mother or a lactation consultant. The most common reason for "not having enough milk" is lack of time to put the baby to the breast, or a baby who, for various reasons, isn't interested. This may be because they are unwell or just too fond of sleeping.

## THE FIRST FEW DAYS

During the last few weeks of pregnancy and in the first two days after birth, your breasts produce around 1 ounce a day of a fluid called colostrum. Colostrum is thicker than mature human milk because it's low in water content and rich in proteins that prime your baby's immune system and protect them from infection in the first months of life. In the days after birth, gradually the amount of lactose sugar and fat in colostrum increases, so that by the end of the first week, the fluid produced looks like milk as we know it. But it takes another two weeks of breastfeeding to produce milk that has the full complement of constituents that characterize "mature" human milk.

## THE AVERAGE NUTRITIONAL COMPOSITION OF MATURE HUMAN MILK

| COMPONENT | PER 4 OUNCES |
| --- | --- |
| Energy (cal) | 79 |
| Protein (g) | 1.5 |
| Fat (g) | 4.9 |
| Carbohydrates (g) | 8.2 |
| Sodium (mg) | 18 |
| Calcium (mg) | 41 |
| Phosphorus (mg) | 18 |
| Iron ( mg) | 89 |
| Vitamin A ( mcg) | 71 |
| Vitamin C (mg) | 4.5 |
| Vitamin D ( mcg) | 0.01 |

Colostrum is rich in proteins that protect your baby from infection in the first months of life.

Breast milk also contains a rich collection of substances that are unique to human milk and ideal for human babies. Many of these substances are relatively resistant to breakdown by digestive enzymes, so they protect the full length of the digestive tract as well the upper respiratory tract. A fully breastfed baby is less likely to develop gastroenteritis, respiratory illnesses (colds) and otitis media (ear infection).

### PROTECTIVE FACTORS IN HUMAN MILK

- » Carbohydrates that prevent pathogens* from attaching to body surfaces
- » Sugars that promote the growth of beneficial bacteria in the lower part of the digestive tract
- » Antibodies known as immunoglobulins (IgA and IgG) that prevent binding and multiplication of pathogens
- » Anti-inflammatory agents
- » Antioxidants
- » White blood cells
- » Lactoferrin, a protein that binds iron and inhibits bugs that need iron for their growth
- » Lysosyme, an enzyme that attacks pathogens
- » Antivirals and other agents that prevent infections

### FEEDING YOUR BABY

Breastfeeding is very cheap and convenient—no mixing, no warming and you can't forget to pack it. It's also good for you, and the perfect food for baby as long as you are well enough and there are no contraindications, such as chemotherapy or certain drugs. For many reasons, experts recommend full breastfeeding (no other sources of food) for the first four to six months of life (see next page).

There is some research that suggests breastfed babies have a lower risk of becoming overweight or obese as they grow older, although the evidence is mixed and not yet conclusive. Being breastfed might also reduce your baby's risk of developing allergies or celiac disease (an allergy to gluten, the protein in wheat, rye and barley) or diabetes (both

---

* A pathogen is a dangerous bacteria or virus that causes disease in humans.

type 1 and type 2) in the future. If you developed gestational diabetes, then breastfeeding may lower your own chances of having type 2 diabetes down the track.

BENEFITS OF BREASTFEEDING
» Protects your baby from illness and infection
» Provides the correct food for your growing baby
» Reduces risk of SIDS
» Reduces diabetes risk (type 1 and type 2)
» Reduces the risk of allergies and asthma
» Is less expensive and more convenient—no need for expensive infant formula and feeding equipment—no washing, sterilizing or preparing
» Reduces your risk of breast and ovarian cancer
» Reduces your risk of postpartum depression
» Reduces your risk of type 2 diabetes if you had gestational diabetes.

Some women are unable to breastfeed for long (for example, they must return to work) or choose not to, but there's no need to feel guilty. Breast milk substitutes are specially formulated to support the healthy growth of young infants. Cow's milk by itself is unsuitable because the concentration of protein and other substances is too high (calves double their weight in one month; a human baby takes three or more months to do so). In past centuries, thousands of babies died from dehydration and kidney failure because full-strength cow's milk was their sole source of food. Babies fed infant formula today grow a little faster than babies fed breast milk, and they may suffer from slightly more infections in the first month of life, but if the infant formula is correctly prepared according to the manufacturer's instructions, we should respect a mother's informed decision to use it.

## BREAST MILK NUTRITION: THE HUMAN MILK FACTORY

In well-nourished women, there's no real connection between your diet and your ability to produce milk. Most mothers will draw on stores built up during pregnancy to supply the building blocks of human milk. Unless they are starving, even undernourished women in poor nations generally produce about 24 ounces of milk per day. But once you introduce formula feedings or solid foods, your milk production will fall to 10–20 ounces a day (the law of supply and demand).

From day to day, whatever you eat, the major macronutrients— protein, fat, carbs—in your milk will remain surprisingly constant. Its calorie yield will be about 60–70 calories per 3.4 ounces. But some micronutrients (vitamins and minerals) will be influenced by the quality of your diet.

## PROTEIN IN HUMAN MILK

Compared with the milk of other mammals, human milk has a very low protein concentration, about 1 gram per 3.4 ounces (see the box on page 123). By six months, it's even less. About 60 percent of the proteins are caseins and 40 percent are whey proteins, which is very different from the ratio in cow's milk (mostly caseins). The proteins in human milk supply all the essential amino acids for building new tissues, hormones and enzymes in your infant. They also protect against infection, help the synthesis of milk sugar (lactose) and carry some of the minerals your baby needs.

## FAT IN HUMAN MILK

Fat is the most variable component of human milk. It provides not only energy but also serves to carry the fat-soluble vitamins and hormones. In well-nourished women, fat averages about 4 grams per 3.4 ounces. Interestingly, the higher the mother's body fat level, the higher the level of fat in their milk. What's more, the nature of the fat in your diet is reflected in your milk. If you consume the long chain omega-3 fats found in many fish, then your milk will also be high in these special fats. They are special because they appear to affect brain development and vision. Evolutionary scientists believe that our very large and complex brain (three times the weight of a chimpanzee's) would not have developed without a rich supply of these fats. These days, we don't eat as much seafood, and it may be difficult to derive enough from other foods.

For this reason, some authorities recommend that lactating moms take a daily fish oil supplement. However, others encourage us to improve the quality of our diets and consume our omega-3 from sources such as fresh and canned fish and omega-3 rich eggs (see the nutrition guide on page 44).

## CARBOHYDRATES IN HUMAN MILK

The main carbohydrate in milk is a sugar called lactose that is similar in structure to table sugar (sucrose) but not as sweet to taste. Interestingly, human milk has the highest concentrations of lactose of any mammal's, with around 7 grams per 3.4 ounces at peak lactation, almost double that of cow's milk (4 grams per 3.4 ounces). One of the reasons for the high concentration may be the glucose requirements of our energy-hungry brain. Lactose is digested by the enzyme lactase found in the cells that line the digestive tract. All of us have sufficient lactase to digest lactose until three to five years of age, after which it undergoes a genetically determined decline in the majority of people. In fact, all mammals (including dogs, cats, rats, mice, etc.) show this decrease. It means that many adults are "lactose-intolerant," showing symptoms such as abdominal distension and even diarrhea if they consume a lot of lactose in one sitting. Fascinatingly, people of Northern European descent have evolved to maintain high levels of lactase throughout life, perhaps because it was a selective advantage at one time to be able to consume more milk.

There is another form of carbohydrate in human milk that is often overlooked, even though there may be as much as 1 gram per 3.4 ounces (more than the weight of protein). Called "oligosaccharides," they are complex sugars that remain undigested in the small intestine, but discourage pathogens in the small intestine and facilitate the growth of friendly bacteria in your baby's large bowel. The beneficial bacteria produce substances that inhibit pathogens and encourage a healthy large intestine. The oligosaccharides in human milk may be another reason that breastfed babies suffer less gastrointestinal disease. Some enterprising manufacturers of breast-milk substitutes now add some form of oligosaccharides to their formulas.

## VITAMIN AND MINERALS IN HUMAN MILK

The concentrations of water-soluble vitamins (vitamin C, $B_1$, $B_2$, $B_6$, etc.) in your milk are directly linked to your current intake of these vitamins. It's one of the best reasons to consume a healthy diet throughout lactation. The fat-soluble vitamins (A, D, E and K) are more constant and are mainly determined by your body stores (usually in the liver). It means that any short-term deficits won't affect the levels in your milk. The concentrations of minerals also appear to be unaffected by your short-term intake. However, it means that if you don't eat well, your stores are being depleted as lactation progresses. Your next baby may not be as well off if you neglect your own needs during this important stage of life.

## NUTRITION RECOMMENDATIONS DURING LACTATION

The energy cost of lactation depends largely on how much milk your baby is drinking. Assuming that human milk provides about 20 calories per ounce, and that you are producing 34 ounces a day, that's a whopping 680 calories in the milk itself. But there's an energy "tax" in making all this milk, so, in fact, you need to ingest an extra 884 calories/day. However, most women have stored some extra fat during pregnancy that they want to lose during the first few months of their baby's life. Allowing for this, the science suggests you need to ingest about 400 to 500 *extra* calories a day—about 20 percent more than usual. Most women just eat more, but some women do less physical activity than usual.

If you entered pregnancy being overweight, then now's a good time to lose those extra pounds. You should do it slowly. Losses of approximately one pound a week do not seem to affect milk production or your baby's rate of growth. If you started pregnancy underweight, then make sure you eat three meals a day and are not losing weight. If your appetite is poor, then make an extra effort to eat small, energy dense healthy snacks (for example, nuts and dried fruit) between meals.

During lactation, you'll need an extra 15–20 g of protein a day—that's relatively easy to obtain in our diet. Nutrients that may be deficient in women who are breastfeeding include folate, calcium and vitamins E,

D and B$_6$. You'll need about 130 micrograms more folate a day than you did pre-pregnancy. (You'll recall from Chapter 3 that many women don't consume enough folate to meet the needs of pregnancy, and folate supplements are routinely advised.) While a supplement is not necessary during lactation, make sure you are eating folate-rich foods—leafy green vegetables being one of the richest sources.

There's about 250–300 mg of calcium in 34 ounces of human milk, equivalent to an extra serving of dairy or dairy alternative per day.

Human milk provides small amounts of vitamin D, around 50 micrograms per liter. This is drawn from stores in your liver, but these are depleted within eight weeks of birth. You'll recall from Chapter 3 that it's nearly impossible to obtain sufficient vitamin D just from food (even with the ideal diet), so you need to expose your skin to brief periods of sunlight at appropriate times of the day, as outlined on page 48.

## EXTRA REQUIREMENTS FOR LACTATION
**(ABOVE NORMAL NONPREGNANT STATE)**

| | | | |
|---|---|---|---|
| Energy (cal) | 478 | Vitamin B$_6$ (mg) | 0.7 |
| Protein (g) | 15-20 | Vitamin B$_{12}$ (mcg) | 0.4 |
| Fiber (g) | 5 | Folate (mcg) | 100 |
| Water as fluid (ml) | 500 | Vitamin C (mg) | 40 |
| Vitamin A (mcg) | 400 | Calcium (mg) | 250–300 |
| Vitamin B$_1$ (mg) | 0.3 | Iodine (mcg) | 120 |
| Vitamin B$_2$ (mg) | 0.5 | Iron (mg) | -9 |
| Niacin (mg) | 3.0 | Zinc (mg) | 4 |
| Omega-3 fats: ALA (mg) | 400 | Omega-3 fats: EPA + DHA (mg) | 55 |

## BREASTFEEDING SNACKS

As discussed above, if you are breastfeeding, your energy and nutrients needs are greater at this time. You can easily meet these needs with a healthy diet, but it may take some extra planning and organization now that you have other responsibilities taking up your time. In Part 4, we give you plenty of practical ideas to ensure you are getting all the nutrients you need, and in Part 5, we provide a selection of quick and tasty recipes to make it easier to put these guidelines into practice.

If you are struggling to find time to eat, preparing a snack and something to drink (a glass of water) ahead of time, so it is ready when you sit down to feed baby, is a good option. It also makes sure you are refueling and rehydrating as baby takes his or her nourishment from you.

## TOP BREASTFEEDING SNACKS

» Whole grain toast or raisin toast
» Whole grain sandwiches
» Glass of milk or soy milk
» Fruit smoothie
» Yogurt
» Dried fruit and nut mix
» Whole grain crispbreads with cheese or avocado and tomato
» Hummus or tzatziki dip with vegetable crudités
» Muesli or oatmeal with low-fat milk or soy milk
» Roasted chickpeas

## CAUTIONS
Some women are at risk of not getting adequate nutrition during lactation.
» Women with highly restricted eating
» Women following a strict vegetarian (or vegan) diet
» Women who are dieting to lose weight
» Women who avoid dairy products
» Women on a very low income.

Vitamin $B_{12}$ deficiency has been reported in the babies of vegetarian moms. A lack of this vitamin can affect neurological development, so ensuring an adequate intake from fortified foods or a supplement is essential. Vitamin D and calcium status may also be low. Judicious sunlight exposure is recommended to stimulate vitamin D synthesis in the skin.

Professional nutrition counseling is recommended in breastfeeding women with type 1 diabetes. Hyperglycemia, hypoglycemia, feeding frequency, mastitis and blood glucose control will all influence insulin requirements.

## FOODS TO LIMIT OR AVOID DURING LACTATION

There are some foods and fluids that are best avoided or limited when you are breastfeeding:

**Caffeine** It is recommended that breastfeeding women limit their caffeine intake to 300 milligrams per day (the amount found in around three cups of coffee). Any caffeine you consume will cross into your breast milk, with the highest levels found around 60 minutes after you have consumed it. Newborns metabolize caffeine very slowly, so the levels can build up if you drink a lot. Remember that caffeine isn't just found in coffee but also tea, cola drinks, energy drinks and chocolate. See the table on page 52 for the caffeine content of common drinks and foods.

**Alcohol** It is best to avoid alcohol while breastfeeding, as alcohol will pass through into your breast milk. If you do choose to drink, wait until your baby has a predictable feeding pattern so you can time any alcohol consumption to minimize the alcohol in your breast milk, remembering that it takes around two hours for your body to metabolize the alcohol in one standard drink. If you have an occasion when you plan to have more than one or two drinks, consider expressing some breast milk beforehand to give your baby while you have alcohol in your system.

**Mercury and other heavy metals** In pregnancy, there are formal recommendations on fish intake, but there are no such restrictions while lactating. In fact, infants are likely to be exposed to higher levels of heavy metals such as mercury before birth than during breastfeeding. Nonetheless, any metals that contaminate drinking water will also be found in breast milk. Formula feeding doesn't solve the problem. Indeed, estimated intake of cadmium (an extremely toxic heavy metal) in powdered formula has been estimated at six times higher than average levels from breast milk. An infant's exposure to cadmium from soy infant formula is about twenty times higher than the levels generally found in breast milk.

**Herbal supplements** If you plan to take any form of supplement when breastfeeding, it is important to ask about its safety and to avoid anything that is not safe while breastfeeding your child. For further information, contact the National Center for Complementary and Alternative Medicine at (888) 644-6226.

## POTENTIAL ALLERGENS

There is no convincing evidence that avoiding certain foods while breastfeeding will reduce the chances of allergy in your child. Although several studies indicate that maternal avoidance of potential food allergens (milk, eggs and fish) while breastfeeding may reduce the risk of atopic eczema in the first years of life, other studies do not confirm this. A review of the research to date concluded there may be some benefits, but further studies were needed.

Some mothers have weaned their babies from breast milk to a hypoallergenic (low allergenicity) formula in the mistaken assumption that this may reduce the risk of allergy in their baby. However, thanks to a large, definitive study conducted in Melbourne, we now know that this is not at all helpful. In that study, children from families with a history of allergy were randomly assigned to hypoallergenic formula or a normal cow's-milk-based formula after they were weaned. After seven years of follow-up, there was absolutely no difference in childhood eczema, asthma or hayfever between the groups. Families at high risk of allergy should, therefore, continue to be encouraged to breastfeed for the many known benefits associated with breastfeeding.

**Smoking** The harmful effect of smoking during pregnancy is well recognized but less is known about how it affects your breastfed baby. If you quit smoking at the start of pregnancy, then there are plenty of reasons to remain a nonsmoker after birth. Babies of smoking moms have a higher incidence of colds, ear infections, asthma and colic during the first months of life. Sudden infant death syndrome (SIDS) is also more common among families in which one or both parents smoke. However, if despite your best efforts, you can't kick the habit, it's still okay to breastfeed. Indeed, your breast milk will help protect your baby from some of the adverse effects of toxins in smoke. Make sure you keep your baby away from secondhand smoke, asking family members and friends to smoke outdoors.

## DEALING WITH COMMON BREASTFEEDING PROBLEMS

Unfortunately, breastfeeding doesn't always go smoothly. The good news is that if you have difficulties, you are not alone and there is help available. Here are some useful tips for dealing with some of the more common problems that can arise.

## TOO MUCH MILK

Some women find they seem to have an oversupply of milk and their babies have trouble coping with the flow. Early on, swollen overfull breasts (engorgement) are the norm, yet this is only temporary and can be resolved with appropriate help. You can expect it to take as much as six weeks for the breasts to adjust to producing the right amount of milk at each feeding. Occasionally, a mother may have continuing problems. La Leche League International is a source of good advice: llli.org.

## NOT ENOUGH MILK

A common assumption is that an unsettled baby is a sign that you might not be producing enough milk. But, just as your body was able to provide everything your baby needed to grow in utero, it is more than capable of producing ex utero. There may be other reasons why your baby is fussing or crying, and you might want to check with your doctor if you have concerns. La Leche League has suggestions to help you discover if your supply really is low, and some tips to help you make more.

If your new baby shows *two or more* of these signs, then you most likely have enough milk:
- At least five wet disposable diapers (or six to eight very wet cloth diapers) in twenty-four hours. Small quantities of strong, dark urine indicate that the baby is in need of more breast milk.
- A very young baby will usually have two or more soft bowel movements a day for several weeks. An older baby may have fewer than this.
- Your baby has good skin color and muscle tone.
- Your baby is alert and reasonably contented and does not constantly want to feed.

- Your baby will probably wake for night feedings. Only a few babies sleep through the night at an early age, while most will wake one or more times during the night for quite some time.
- Some weight gain and growth in length and head circumference.

For more advice on this topic, go to llli.org/nb/nbmilksupplyissues.html.

## MASTITIS

Mastitis is usually the result of a blocked milk duct. Some of the milk behind the blocked duct is forced into nearby breast tissue, causing it to become inflamed. The inflammation is called mastitis (or "milk fever"). Infection may or may not be present. Symptoms can come on quickly and make you feel as if you are getting the flu, such as shivering and aches and pains. The breast may become sore, red and swollen, even hot and painful. See your doctor urgently. It's best to start treatment as soon as you feel a lump or sore spot in your breast.

Importantly, this is *not* the time to wean. Your breasts should be kept as empty as possible, and your baby's sucking is the best way to achieve this. The milk is quite safe for your baby to drink. For more advice on dealing with mastitis, go to llli.org/faq/mastitis.html.

## BREAST AND NIPPLE CARE

Most new mothers find their nipples become a little sore or tender at the beginning of lactation. Make sure your bra is a proper fitting maternity bra that accommodates your newly endowed frame (sorry ladies—this is not the time to wear your sexy bras). Don't use anything on your nipples that might dry out your skin, such as an alcohol gel. Avoid scrubbing with rough towels or brushes.

During feedings, make sure baby is properly positioned at and attached to the breast. (Remember there's an art to breastfeeding. Seek advice from nursing staff or a lactation consultant on attaching your baby to the breast when first attempting to breastfeed.) Offer the less sore side first. When baby has had enough, gently break suction with a clean finger. Express a few drops of your hindmilk and smear on the nipple. You might like to leave your bra open for a few minutes until your nipples are dry. If you use nursing pads, change frequently. Use breast shells or nipple protectors over tender nipples to stop clothes from rubbing and allow air to circulate.

## Lactation consultants

La Leche League International has been helping women master the art of breastfeeding through mother-to-mother support, encouragement, information and education for more than fifty years. It has chapters all over the country led by experienced mothers who have breastfed their own babies and who have been trained and accredited by La Leche League International to help mothers and mothers-to-be with all aspects of breastfeeding. For more details and to find a La Leche League chapter near you, visit llli.org. You can also ask your doctor to recommend a local consultant.

## WHEN BREASTFEEDING ISN'T POSSIBLE

Sometimes it's just not possible to begin breastfeeding soon after birth. Some babies are born prematurely and need to be placed in incubators for days or even months. There may be other complications or factors, such as chemotherapy or drugs that you need to take, but not your baby (via breast milk). *Don't stress.* Thousands of babies worldwide are fed breast-milk substitutes, including ones designed especially for premature babies. If you wish, you can use a breast-milk pump to collect your milk and give it to your baby via a tube or bottle. You can even begin lactation at a later date.

## UNDERSIZE AND PREMATURE BABIES NEED SPECIAL CARE

Infants that are born full-term are able to feed from the breast or bottle without much trouble. However, it's common for babies that are born preterm to have initial difficulties with sucking and swallowing. They may require tube feeding until they are old enough and medically stable enough to feed normally. Even then, they may be a little weak and uncoordinated—it's harder than you think to suck, breathe and swallow. If you have a premature baby, it's important that you have individual professional help, so your baby gains weight and catches up without complications. Problems with feeding now can spell long-term problems that you want to avoid, such as poor physical and motor development.

## GETTING YOUR FIGURE BACK

It is normal for your postdelivery weight to be higher than your pre-conception weight. Your uterus is still bigger (and will gradually shrink), your blood volume is still higher and nature ensures you have 7–10 pounds of fat stores to facilitate breastfeeding. If you have retained extra weight after your pregnancy, following a strict diet with the promise of getting your figure back quickly might be tempting. However, restrictive diets and rapid weight loss are not recommended even after baby arrives, and this is particularly important if you are breastfeeding. Your energy and nutrient needs are higher at this time, and dieting may affect your milk production, not to mention your energy levels, which are already likely to be suffering with the demands of a newborn baby and lack of sleep. Even if you are not breastfeeding, unless you can sustain the changes you make, your weight-loss results are likely to be short-lived. It is much better to focus on making sustainable changes to your eating and exercise habits—changes you can see yourself maintaining in the long term. This is even more important now that you are a parent, as you want to be a good role model for your child.

## EXERCISE POST-PREGNANCY

Health professionals encourage a gradual resumption of exercising after your baby is born. Some may ask you to wait until your six-week postpartum checkup. Generally, if you exercised throughout your pregnancy and had a normal vaginal delivery, you can safely perform your pregnancy workout (see Chapter 6) or at least light exercise, such as walking, modified push-ups and stretching, within days of giving birth. Depending on the nature of your delivery, your obstetric-care provider can offer specific advice. Make sure it's a gentle start. After your first postpartum week, take a slow to moderate 30-minute walk three times a week. As you regain strength, you can increase the length or number of walks. If you had a Caesarean section, expect to wait about six to eight weeks to exercise. However, walking at an easy pace is encouraged, because it promotes healing and helps prevent complications such as blood clots.

If you weren't active during your pregnancy, or tapered off your fitness routine as the weeks went on, start slow and check with your doctor or midwife before you begin. In any case, remember that your joints and ligaments will still be loose for about three to five months. If you want to take an exercise class, try to find one taught by a postpartum exercise specialist or go for a low-impact class focused on toning and stretching.

As a parent it can be difficult to find time for yourself to exercise, and for many, starting a family can signal the end of a regular exercise program. With babies and toddlers, walking with a stroller is the best way for you to stay active (and can be a good way to get your little one to sleep!), or join a mother-and-baby exercise class. As your child/children get older, try being active together as a family—this will give you the benefit of spending time together, maintaining your own fitness and encouraging your kids to be active. Limiting sedentary time, including screen time, for the whole family is also important.

Many fitness centers, gyms and yoga studios offer exercise classes for new moms.

Exercise is good for you, but in the first few months after you give birth, don't overdo it. Your body may need time to heal, and you need time to adjust to your new role and to care for and bond with your baby.

# FREQUENTLY ASKED QUESTIONS

**"Is it safe to lose weight while I am breastfeeding?"**

Part of the weight you gain during pregnancy will be extra fat stores for breastfeeding. It is, therefore, normal to lose some weight while breastfeeding, although some women will lose weight soon after their baby is born and others not until they finish breastfeeding. It is actually good to lose this extra weight, particularly if you have subsequent pregnancies, as gaining a bit with each baby and not losing it can make it much harder to return to a healthy weight later on. Having said that, you should aim for a gradual weight loss of no more than about one pound per week. You can achieve this with a healthy eating plan and regular exercise. Avoid rapid weight loss and restrictive diets that are unlikely to provide the nutrients you and your baby need and may affect breast milk production. If you feel as if you need to lose weight more quickly, you should speak to your doctor and get the help of a registered dietitian (RD) who can help you plan a weight loss diet suitable for breastfeeding.

**"I'm losing too much weight—what do I do?"**

While many mothers are thinking about how they can lose their pregnancy weight, not everyone has this problem. Particularly if you were a healthy weight or underweight prior to pregnancy, or someone who loses weight easily, then breastfeeding may cause your weight to drop off too quickly. If this is the case, try to increase the size of your meals and include regular nutritious snacks between meals. While it can be tempting to fill up on foods high in saturated fat and sugar (such as cookies and chocolate), it is best to choose more nutrient-dense snacks to ensure you are getting all the nutrients you and your baby need, as well as the extra calories needed to prevent weight loss. Good choices include dried fruit and nuts, whole grain toast with peanut butter or avocado, fruit smoothies and yogurt. You could also seek out calorie-dense fluids such as milk, soy milk or fruit juice in place of water.

## POSTPARTUM DEPRESSION—YOU ARE NOT ALONE

It's no surprise that adjusting to motherhood can be difficult. In fact, for many women, having a baby is the most significant life-changing event they will ever experience. Coping with the day-to-day demands of a new baby can precipitate depression or anxiety in some women, particularly if these have occurred in the past. It's more than just a low mood—it's a serious illness.

In the United States, around one in eight moms experiences postpartum depression (PPD)—depression that usually occurs in the first three months after having a baby but can happen any time within the first year. Anxiety is also more common during this time, and the first signs may even occur during the latter half of pregnancy. While everyone feels sad, moody or low from time to time, some of us experience these feelings intensely, for long periods of time and often without reason. Mothers with depression find it hard to function every day, and find even the activities they used to enjoy have lost their attraction. Everything seems like too much trouble. It's important to acknowledge your feelings and speak up so that you can get the help you need to tackle your depression. For more information, we recommend the Postpartum Support International website and the Mayo Clinic: mayoclinic.com/health/postpartum-depression/DS00546.

The Mayo Clinic offers these suggestions if you have PPD:

» **Seek professional help from a doctor or psychologist.**

» **Make healthy lifestyle choices.** Include physical activity, such as a walk with your baby, in your daily routine. Eat healthy foods and avoid alcohol.

» **Set realistic expectations.** Don't pressure yourself to do everything. Scale back your expectations for the perfect household. Do what you can and leave the rest. Ask for help when you need it.

» **Make time for yourself.** If you feel like the world is coming down around you, take some time for yourself. Get dressed, leave the house and visit a friend or run an errand. Or schedule some time alone with your partner.

» **Respond positively.** When faced with a negative situation, focus on keeping your thoughts positive. Even if an unwanted situation doesn't change, you can change the way you think and behave in response to it—a brief course of cognitive behavioral therapy may help you learn how to do this.

» **Avoid isolation.** Talk with your partner, family and friends about how you're feeling. Ask other mothers about their experiences. Ask your doctor about local support groups for new moms or women who have postpartum depression.

## ARE YOU DEPRESSED?

**The Edinburgh Postnatal Depression Scale** is a set of questions designed to see if a new mother may have depression. The answers *will not provide a diagnosis*—for that you need to see a doctor or other health professional. However, the answers will tell you if you, or someone close to you, has symptoms that are common in women with PPD (known as postnatal depression, or PND, in countries such as the United Kingdom and Australia).

## The Edinburgh Postnatal Depression Scale

To complete this set of questions, mothers should circle the number next to the response that comes closest to how they have felt *in the past seven days.*

**1.  I have been able to laugh and see the funny side of things.**
- 0   As much as I always could
- 1   Not quite so much now
- 2   Definitely not so much now
- 3   Not at all

**2.  I have looked forward with enjoyment to things.**
- 0   As much as I ever did
- 1   Rather less than I used to
- 2   Definitely less than I used to
- 3   Hardly at all

**3.  I have blamed myself unnecessarily when things went wrong.**
- 3   Yes, most of the time
- 2   Yes, some of the time
- 1   Not very often
- 0   No, never

**4.  I have been anxious or worried for no good reason.**
- 0   No, not at all
- 1   Hardly ever
- 2   Yes, sometimes
- 3   Yes, very often

**5. I have felt scared or panicky for no very good reason.**

- 3 Yes, quite a lot
- 2 Yes, sometimes
- 1 No, not much
- 0 No, not at all

**6. Things have been getting on top of me.**

- 3 Yes, most of the time I haven't been able to cope at all
- 2 Yes, sometimes I haven't been coping as well as usual
- 1 No, most of the time I have coped quite well
- 0 No, I have been coping as well as ever

**7. I have been so unhappy that I have had difficulty sleeping.**

- 3 Yes, most of the time
- 2 Yes, sometimes
- 1 Not very often
- 0 No, not at all

**8. I have felt sad or miserable.**

- 3 Yes, most of the time
- 2 Yes, quite often
- 1 Not very often
- 0 No, not at all

**9. I have been so unhappy that I have been crying.**

- 3 Yes, most of the time
- 2 Yes, quite often
- 1 Only occasionally
- 0 No, never

**10. The thought of harming myself has occurred to me.**

- 3 Yes, quite often
- 2 Sometimes
- 1 Hardly ever
- 0 Never

The total score is calculated by adding together the numbers circled for each of the ten items. The higher the score, the more likely it is that the person completing the questionnaire is distressed and may be depressed.

Note: Scores provide only a rough guide as to whether a woman has PPD. For a full diagnosis, it is important to see a doctor. Cox, Holden and Sagovsky, *British Journal of Psychiatry, 1987.*

# Chapter 9

# Weaning your baby

Weaning means different things to different people. To many people, weaning is the period during which our babies come to have fewer and fewer breastfeedings until they are completely nourished by other foods and drinks—that is, fully weaned. To some, it is the simple process of introducing foods other than milk to your baby's diet. To others, it means introducing formula in a bottle or sippy cup to a breastfed baby. Whatever it means to you, the time to wean your baby is when you or your baby decides that it is right, taking into account the needs of your baby, you and your home and family situation. Well-meaning friends and relatives should not be part of the decision-making. If you are undecided about what to do, then perhaps a chat with your local La Leche League group leader may help.

Breast milk by itself contains all the nourishment needed to promote healthy growth and development in babies for the first six months of life. While babies begin to have other foods and drinks from about four to six months onward, breast milk is still the major part of the growing baby's diet. No matter how long you continue to breastfeed, your milk is always nutritious and absolutely right for your baby's stage of development.

Slowly reducing the number of breastfeedings further protects your baby during the weaning period. Although you are making less and less milk, your baby is still receiving added protection from the milk you do produce. Breast milk contains more antibodies to bacterial and viral diseases as weaning progresses. This is one of its many benefits and ensures that your baby is protected while being introduced to new foods and exploring new surroundings. Whenever weaning from the breast begins, try to make it gradual. It is best not to set a time limit so that both of you (and your breasts) adjust gradually.

For more information, go to llli.org/nb/nbweaning.html.

## STARTING SOLIDS

Starting solid foods is a new stage in your baby's development, but it also brings lots of questions: When should my baby start solids? What foods do I use? How much? Does it mean I have to stop breastfeeding? Every baby and family is different.

Importantly, babies don't benefit from starting solids or foods other than milk or formula before four to six months of age. Up until then, they have a natural tongue-thrust reflex that makes them push out their tongue when food is put in their mouth. They do not need the extra calories that solid foods may give them. Your baby's kidneys are not designed to excrete the large amount of salt found in most processed foods. Research also shows that a baby will not sleep any longer when solids are started. Babies wake for many reasons, of which hunger may only be one.

Somewhere around four to six months, your baby will let you know when he or she is ready for extra foods. For example, they may try to take food from your plate (or somebody else's) or show interest in eating when you do. Make suitable foods available and let your baby decide what they want.

You may be worried about your baby's intake of iron. Research has shown that the risk of low iron is small in healthy full-term babies still exclusively breastfed between six and twelve months. It is a good idea to offer foods that contain iron, such as cereals like quinoa and oatmeal, as one of their first foods. Other good iron sources, such as meat, legumes and tofu, can be introduced around eight months of age.

Let your baby set the pace. There is no point in forcing or coaxing your baby to eat. Just be willing to give help when it is needed. Always stop when your baby does not want any more. Their appetite is the best guide to their needs. The amount taken at first may be quite tiny— perhaps only a quarter of a teaspoon—but once they get the idea, your baby may eat one or more teaspoons of a well-liked food. At this stage, solids are a learning activity for your baby—learning about tastes and textures—and breast milk will still be meeting their nutritional needs.

Don't worry if your baby does not like some foods. No single food is essential to the diet. There are always other choices.

Be aware of the possibility of choking and always stay with your baby while they are eating or chewing. Wait for a few days after introducing each new food before introducing another. Reactions to new foods may include a rash or eczema, diarrhea or constipation, or your baby crying more than usual, maybe from a tummy ache. An allergic reaction usually occurs right after the food is eaten or even touches the baby's skin, but other reactions may take two to three days to occur. Spacing out new foods will help you figure out which food caused a reaction if one does happen.

It used to be thought that some foods should be delayed until a baby is nine to twelve months or older, to reduce the risk of the child developing food allergies. Recent research has shown that this does not reduce the allergy risk, even for babies from families with a history of allergies. Experts currently advise that almost any food, including eggs, wheat and fish, can be introduced from six months onward. It is now thought that small amounts given often from about six months of age, particularly while still breastfeeding, help to reduce allergies rather than cause them. If there is a family history of nut allergy, your health practitioner should be consulted. Because nuts can cause a choking hazard, wait until your baby has good chewing skills (usually after eighteen months of age) to introduce them.

## FIRST FOOD IDEAS

**Fruit** (from six months) Mashed banana, ripe pear or avocado; unsweetened puréed cooked apple or other fruit; fruit purée mixed with cereal. Many babies also love summer fruits like peaches, mango, watermelon and cantaloupe.

**Vegetables** (from six months) Baked or steamed sweet potato, white potato, squash or carrot; dried peas or beans, soaked and boiled until soft, or baked beans from a can (choose the no-salt-added type), mashed or puréed; any cooked vegetable, mashed or puréed if necessary.

**Meat, including chicken** (from seven to eight months) Meat scraped to a pulp with a knife, wrapped in foil and steamed or baked; grilled meat cut up finely, or you can use a blender.

**Soups** Cooled homemade soups based on stocks that have had the fat skimmed; vegetables can be puréed into the stock and, later, small pieces can be left in the soup for your baby to chew.

**Fish** (from seven to eight months) Any cooked fish without bones.

**Wheat-based cereals** (from seven to eight months).

**Milk products** (from nine to ten months) Yogurt, cottage cheese or homemade pudding.

**Eggs** (from seven to eight months) Soft-boiled eggs scooped out of the shell and mixed with fresh bread crumbs; poached or scrambled eggs.

**Pasta** Larger shapes of well-cooked pasta are fun as first foods. Cool before offering.

**Baby rice cereal** (from six months) Mixed with breast milk, formula or boiled water, cooled and puréed with fruit and vegetables.

## SOME IDEAS FOR FINGER FOODS

**Fruit** Piece of banana; peeled and cored apple or pear. Grated apple or other fruit; pieces of melon or papaya (without seeds); an orange quarter, minus peel and seeds; stone fruit with stone removed.

**Meat or alternative** A small amount of cooled meat on a safe bone, neither sharp nor brittle, for example, lamb chop; slices of homemade meat loaf; firm tofu cooked in long thin slices.

**Fish** Cooled homemade fish sticks; flakes of cooked, cooled fish with every bone removed.

**Vegetables, for babies with teeth** A piece of raw peeled celery or other salad vegetables; fresh, raw, or cooked green stringless beans; grated raw carrot; slices of cooked potato, carrot or other vegetable.

**Bread** Preferably low GI whole grain if baby is over nine months; homemade biscuits (bake thick slices or crusts in a very low oven until they are quite crisp and dry); toast, plain or buttered; sandwiches.

**Pasta** Boiled and cooled pasta shapes.

**Cheese** Cheese sticks; grated cheese.

**Eggs** Pieces of hard-boiled egg yolk or whole egg; strips of omelet.

Often the best food for your baby is the meal you are preparing for the rest of the family, adapted for your baby.

## BUILDING GOOD EATING HABITS FROM THE START

Children have evolved to mimic their parents' behavior, and they are watching you more carefully than you would ever know. If you eat it, they will want to also. If you eat a balanced diet, they will, too. Being a good role model applies to eating, exercising and all aspects of your behavior, and food habits that are adopted early on are difficult to alter later. If you flavor everything with salt, they will grow to prefer salty food. If you over-sweeten, then they expect food to taste extremely sweet. If you expect them to eat *everything* on their plate, then they learn to ignore internal satiety signals. They will learn to eat until they feel uncomfortably full. It's no surprise then to find they are overweight early on.

But it's not easy in today's world to confine your children's food intake to only the healthiest foods. Children's parties are common; family celebrations are occasions that call for special foods. The best way to handle these situations is not to deny your children, but teach them that "party foods" are for parties or about "sometimes" foods. They should not be part of your normal pantry. Ice cream, soft drinks, cookies and cake, French fries and potato chips are all indulgence foods. You might insist that "sometimes" foods only come with some outdoor activity, such as a popcicle at the beach or potato chips at the park. (A little indulgence is a good thing, but make sure it's just that—a *little* indulgence.)

The idea of "sometimes" foods is one that kids seem to easily understand and the expression is now widely used among families.

One of the best ways of teaching your child to love healthy foods is to involve them in the preparation of the meal and even growing vegetables in the garden. Young children can tear up various types of lettuce for a salad (and a little food sampling won't hurt), and when they are old enough, they can help you draw a funny face with carrots, raisins and apple slices. Books dedicated to cooking with children can be a real delight. You'll find it one of the most enjoyable and rewarding ways of spending quality time with your children. By the time they are old enough to be safe in a kitchen, you could insist that your kids prepare at least one family meal a week (no harm in trying!).

## TV VIEWING AND SCREEN TIME

We now know that watching TV for hours on end is the fast track to excess weight. In fact, the more hours we spend being a couch potato, the heavier we are. Some research suggests our metabolic rates drop below that of sleeping during a long period in front of the screen. Watching TV is often coupled with eating mindlessly, making us even more likely to gain extra pounds of body fat. Some family rules that are helpful are:

» No TV during family mealtimes
» No TV in bedrooms
» No more than two hours of TV or screen time per day

## ENCOURAGE FAMILY ACTIVITY

Exercise is important for everyone, and it is a good idea to encourage physical activity from a young age. It can be more difficult to find time to exercise once you have children, so finding activities you can do together as a family means you can maintain your own fitness, encourage your kids to be active and spend quality time together. These are just a few ideas:

» Walk to the local park to play or kick a ball around.
» When possible, walk your kids to school, or park further away and walk part of the way.
» Walk or jog while younger kids ride a bike or scooter alongside you.
» If you have a home video game console, consider buying those games that incorporate some form of exercise or body movement—there are lots of fun activities the whole family can do together.

- » Most kids like music and dancing, so put on your (or their) favorite music and have a home dance party, or consider a dance DVD like Zumba that everyone can try.
- » On warm weekends, walk along the beach, then go for a swim.
- » Consider active outings on holidays and weekends, such as going to the zoo or nature center, or exploring different tourist attractions on foot.

## SUMMARY
## 10 tips for life beyond Due-Day

1. If possible, learn the gentle art of breastfeeding.
2. Introduce appropriate foods at around four to six months of age.
3. Be a good role model—children mimic their parents.
4. Eat well and exercise for your well-being, not for weight loss.
5. Stock your fridge and cupboards with fresh healthy foods.
6. Keep the less-than-healthy options for "sometimes" foods and combine with outdoor activity.
7. Be physically active as a family.
8. Limit screen time—even for babies!
9. Look after your mental health.
10. Be aware of signs of PPD.

# PART 4
# Putting it all on the plate

*We know it's taken us a lot of time to get to this point (what to eat), but we don't apologize. We believe that explaining the science and evidence behind new nutrition recommendations in pregnancy will encourage you to put theory into practice. In Part 4, we show you exactly how you can ensure you are getting all the nutrition you need without gaining excess weight by following the principles of a low GI diet. We describe step by step how to put together healthy meals and snacks that will also tempt your taste buds. We also show you the top food sources of the important nutrients for pre-conception, pregnancy and breastfeeding. And to make life as easy as possible, we have provided a comprehensive pantry guide to help you stock the cupboards.*

# Chapter 10

# The Low GI Eating Plan—putting it into action

Whether you are pregnant or trying to conceive, good nutrition is an essential part of optimizing your own health and that of your unborn child. Eating well prior to conceiving ensures that your body is in the best position to support a pregnancy, while good nutrition during pregnancy is essential to provide the nutrients your baby needs to grow and develop and those you need to stay healthy throughout your pregnancy.

While the benefits are clear, we also know it is easy to get confused about exactly what you should be eating when pregnant or trying to conceive, and those foods you may need to avoid. So in this chapter we outline our eight steps, which explain precisely what you need to eat pre-conception and during pregnancy to meet the nutritional needs of you and your baby while also managing your weight.

# 8

# steps to the Low GI Eating Plan

| | |
|---|---|
| **1** Manage your weight | **2** Focus on nutrient density |
| **3** Eat regularly | **4** Keep your protein lean |
| **5** Be choosy about fats | **6** Be smart about carbs |
| **7** Don't forget fluids | **8** Avoid food hazards |

## STEP 1 Manage your weight

We have covered the issue of weight gain in detail in Chapter 4, so we won't repeat that information here except to say that optimizing your weight before conception, managing your weight gain during pregnancy and getting back to your pre-pregnancy weight after your baby has arrived is important for both you and your baby. This can be achieved by balancing a healthy diet (which we discuss further on the following pages) with regular exercise. Remember this is not a time for restrictive diets or rapid weight loss: Building healthy eating habits and being active should be your goals.

Balance a healthy diet with regular exercise.

# 2 Focus on nutrient density

## WHAT IS "NUTRIENT DENSITY"?

Nutrient density is all about quality over quantity. Nutrient-dense foods are those that contribute greater amounts of beneficial nutrients per calorie to the overall diet. By selecting these foods first, you can obtain all the nutrients you need in your diet without exceeding your energy needs. It is wise for everyone to try to select mostly nutrient-dense foods in order to maximize nutritional intake and manage their weight, but this is particularly important during pregnancy when your need for essential nutrients increases more than your energy (or calorie) needs.

Nutrient-dense foods include fruits, vegetables, legumes, whole grains, nuts, seeds, fish, lean meats and poultry and low-fat dairy products. And it's probably not hard to figure out that the nutrient-poor foods are those such as cookies, cakes, pastries, candy, chips and soft drinks: foods high in energy that provide little in the way of nutrition and are best kept for occasional treats rather than everyday choices.

## HIGH NUTRIENT DENSITY OPTIONS

Foods with a high nutrient density are largely those that tend to be less processed, and most come from the plant kingdom. If they are rich in carbohydrates, they should have a low GI. These include:

**Vegetables and fruit** For maximum nutrition, include a wide variety of different colored fruit and vegetables each day, and make these the basis of your meals and snacks. Aim for two to three servings of fruit each day and at least five servings of vegetables and salads. One serving is a medium-size piece of fruit, half a cup cooked vegetables or one cup of salad. At meals, try to fill half your plate with fruit and vegetables.

**Low GI grains (preferably whole grains)** These provide more nutrients and fiber than highly processed grains, so should be your first choice. Think steel-cut oats; certain whole grain breads; white and whole grain pasta; and low GI, high-fiber breakfast cereals and crispbreads in place of the more processed varieties. You can also experiment with less commonly used grains such as barley, quinoa, cracked wheat and buckwheat. Aim to include at least one serving of whole grains with most meals—for example, oatmeal or muesli at breakfast, a low GI whole grain sandwich or quinoa salad at lunch and barley or noodles with a stir-fry at dinner.

**Legumes** Lentils, chickpeas, kidney beans, cannellini beans, cranberry (or pinto) beans, butter beans, black-eye beans and navy beans are all low GI, nutritious, economical and versatile. The easiest option is to add them to your regular meals—for example, kidney beans in a casserole, lentils in a curry, mashed potatoes with cannellini beans or chickpeas in a stir-fry. You could also include a few vegetarian meals made with legumes such as a lentil shepherd's pie, chickpea and vegetable curry or Mexican bean burritos. Either way, try to include them in your diet a few times per week, or daily if you are vegetarian.

**Nuts and seeds** Although high in fat and energy, nuts and seeds are rich in the healthy fats important for pregnancy, and are packed with a variety of vitamins and minerals, including iron, zinc and magnesium. Add them to meals or eat them as a portable satisfying snack. Nut and seed spreads (such as tahini) are a nutritious alternative to butter.

**Lean protein foods** These include lean meats, poultry, fish, seafood, tofu and eggs. In addition to protein, these foods also supply important vitamins and minerals for pregnancy, including iron, zinc, vitamin $B_{12}$ (animal products only) and omega-3 fats (fish and seafood). Aim to include a small serving of protein (one quarter of your plate) with most meals, although at breakfast this may come from milk, soy milk or yogurt instead.

**Dairy or soy products or alternatives** Milk, soy milk and yogurt provide protein and all important calcium. If choosing soy milk or other milk alternatives such as rice, almond or oat milk, make sure

# Focus on nutrient density

you choose brands with added calcium, and if you are vegetarian, look for one with added vitamin $B_{12}$. Aim to include around three servings of a calcium-rich food each day—if you don't eat dairy products or calcium-fortified alternatives, you will need to incorporate other calcium-rich foods such as hard tofu, almonds, dried figs, unhulled tahini, Asian greens, kale and broccoli.

## THE FOODS TO AVOID: LOW NUTRIENT DENSITY OPTIONS

If these are on your list of favorite foods, you may wonder how you can do without them. You don't necessarily have to cut them all out, but these foods should only make up a small part of your diet and not at the expense of more nutritious foods. Think of them as a treat, a small reward for otherwise eating well and exercising sensibly.

**Cakes, cookies and pastries** These are generally high in sugar, and saturated and trans fats, with little nutritional value. Good alternatives would be a slice of raisin bread or some whole grain toast spread with jam or honey. Of course, you can also make your own healthy cakes and muffins using ingredients like whole wheat flour, oats, fresh or dried fruits, nuts, seeds and healthy oils. We have included some recipes to get you started in Part 5.

**Candy** A combination of sugar, colors and flavors, candy doesn't have much going for it nutritionally. Dried fruit is a great alternative— while still high in natural sugars, dried fruits are packed with nutrition and are a convenient and portable snack that's great for satisfying sweet cravings. Try a few dates with a handful of walnuts or some dried figs and almonds.

**Chocolate** High in fat and sugar, chocolate adds up the calories quickly. Dark chocolate is the best choice, as the antioxidants it contains have some health benefits, and it is also easier to eat in small amounts. If chocolate is something you can't do without, make it a rule to buy only good quality, and enjoy small amounts at any one time.

**Chips and savory snacks** High in salt, saturated fat and, possibly, trans fats, these are also something to put on the occasional list. Better choices include roasted chickpeas or soybeans, plain popcorn or whole grain crackers. Note that rice crackers may be low in fat, but they have a very high GI and are also high in salt.

**Soft drinks, punches, iced teas and fruit juice drinks** These provide a large hit of carbs (around ten teaspoons of sugar in a can of soft drink), but no nutrients to mention. If you don't like plain water, try sparkling mineral water or seltzer with a squeeze of fresh lemon or lime or a few mint leaves. If you want more flavor, try half fruit juice (without added sugar) and half water or sparkling water—although still high in natural sugars, fruit juice does provide some vitamins not found in other sugar-sweetened drinks, so would be a better choice.

# 3 Eat regularly

**STEP**

Eating regularly over the day has benefits for everyone, but particularly if you are pregnant. Eating small regular meals and snacks can help to supply your growing baby with a steady stream of energy and nutrients, manage your appetite, keep your blood glucose levels stable and help with morning sickness and heartburn.

## DON'T SKIP BREAKFAST

Eating breakfast regularly is something we should all do, and this is particularly the case during pregnancy. Remember that your baby is constantly taking energy and nutrients for growth, so fueling up after your overnight fast is important. Eating this meal is also important for maintaining your own energy levels and preventing hunger and snacking on less healthy choices later in the day. Many studies have found that people who eat breakfast regularly have a better overall nutrient intake. A study in pregnant women found that those who ate a cereal for breakfast were much more likely to have an adequate intake of a variety of important vitamins and minerals, including folate, iron, zinc, calcium and vitamins A, C, D and E, as well as fiber.

When it comes to weight control, there is plenty of evidence to show that breakfast eaters are less likely to be overweight. Missing breakfast, on the other hand, has been associated with increased insulin and blood fat levels, and may lead to weight gain. A recent study found that those who skipped breakfast were 34 percent more likely to be obese and had a lower health-related quality of life. Another found that the individuals who skipped breakfast in both childhood and as adults had a larger waist circumference, higher fasting insulin levels and higher levels of total and LDL ("bad") cholesterol compared to those who ate breakfast at both times.

As a parent or soon-to-be parent, you also want to be a good role model when it comes to eating well. Many studies have found that kids who eat breakfast are better able to concentrate at school and may have stronger memories and perform higher on school tests. They are also less likely to be overweight. Interestingly, one study found that children of mothers who skipped breakfast before and during early pregnancy were almost twice as likely to be overweight and three times more likely to be obese at the age of five.

All in all, there are many good reasons to include this important meal, even if it means ten minutes less sleep!

## FREQUENTLY ASKED QUESTIONS

**"I have terrible morning sickness when I wake up and can't face breakfast—do you have any suggestions?"**
Start by taking your time getting out of bed. Sit up slowly and nibble a few dry crackers before you get out of bed—keep these by your bedside so you have them ready when you wake up. If you can rest for a little while before getting out of bed, this can help. The smell of food cooking can worsen nausea, so try to avoid this by sticking to a cold breakfast or getting someone else to prepare it for you. Dry salty foods often work best—for example, a slice of toast. If you can't manage solid food but feel you could drink something, a fruit smoothie or fresh juice would be good options.

## SNACKS COUNT

Snacks are not just something to fill a gap between breakfast and lunch, to pick up your energy levels midafternoon or to satisfy those post-dinner sweet cravings. The right snacks can make a valuable contribution to your eating plan, while choosing less nutritious options can make it much harder to get all the nutrients that you and baby need while also preventing excess weight gain. Good snack choices include fresh or dried fruit, yogurt, nuts, low GI whole grain crackers or toast and low GI raisin bread.

## PLATE MATTERS

The easiest way to get the right balance of nutrients while keeping your weight under control is to focus on your plate at mealtimes. Aim

# 3 Eat regularly

to fill half of your plate with non-starchy vegetables and salads, one-quarter of your plate with grains or starchy vegetables, and the remaining quarter with some lean protein. Add a small amount of healthy fat and some herbs and spices for flavor, and you have the perfect meal! This doesn't need to be an exact science, but if you keep this guide in mind for your lunch and dinner meals, you will be on the right track to eating well during pregnancy.

## FREQUENTLY ASKED QUESTIONS

**"Some days my heartburn is so bad that anything I eat seems to make it worse—what do I do?"**

The best way to manage heartburn is by eating small regular meals and snacks through the day. Make sure you always sit down to eat, take time to chew your food well and relax while eating. Fatty and spicy meals can make heartburn worse as can chocolate, caffeine and alcohol. If none of this helps, then pharmacists can advise on the best antacids for pregnancy. (See tips on page 56 for more details on managing heartburn.)

**"Is it safe to fast while I am pregnant?"**

Fasting is an important part of many religious customs. While there are often exemptions or allowances for pregnant women (such as making up the fast at a later time), some women still choose to fast in pregnancy due to their personal beliefs or religious commitments. While it is best to avoid prolonged periods of fasting while pregnant, this is a personal choice that only you can make, taking into account both you and your baby. If you do decide to fast, it is best to discuss this with your doctor first, particularly if your religion doesn't allow any food or water during the fast. You could also consider other alternatives to fasting, such as only giving up certain food and drinks, or abstaining from other activities you enjoy. Or you could just fast for part of the day rather than the whole day. If you do fast, it is important to stay hydrated, to avoid strenuous activity and to get plenty of rest. If you experience any symptoms such as headaches, feeling faint or dizzy, severe nausea, stomach pains or fatigue, you should see your doctor immediately.

# STEP 4
# Keep your protein lean

Protein is important for many reasons, including the growth and repair of our muscles and cells. While your protein needs increase during pregnancy (you need around 30 percent more than when you are not pregnant) and breastfeeding (you need around 45 percent more), most of us eat much more protein than we need anyway, so meeting these increased requirements isn't difficult if you are consuming enough calories. The amount of protein you need depends on your weight, but the minimum amount for the average woman is around 60 grams per day during the second and third trimesters of pregnancy and around 70 grams per day when breastfeeding. According to a study of protein intake published in the *American Journal of Clinical Nutrition* in 2008, the average American woman eats around 70 grams of protein daily.

In food terms, 60 grams of protein could be obtained by eating a bowl of oatmeal with milk or soy milk at breakfast, a low GI whole grain cheese and salad sandwich at lunch, 3½ ounces of lean meat, chicken or fish with vegetables at dinner, and a 6-ounce container of yogurt and a handful of almonds for snacks. If you are vegetarian, you could replace the meat with 5 ounces of tofu or one cup of lentils, and if you are vegan, replace the cheese at lunch with falafel and the yogurt with soy yogurt.

## THE BEST PROTEIN SOURCES

Protein is found in most foods including meat, poultry, fish, seafood, eggs, tofu and soy foods, dairy products, nuts, seeds and grains. Even vegetables contain small amounts; however, they are not a major contributor to our protein intakes.

Good protein sources include:

**Lean meats** Compared to fatty and processed meats, lean cuts of red meat (such as lean gound beef or steak) provide

# 4 Keep your protein lean

significantly more protein as well as valuable iron, zinc and vitamin B$_{12}$. However, one study found that women who ate more red meat prior to pregnancy were more likely to develop gestational diabetes, and a number of studies have linked high intakes of red meat to type 2 diabetes risk. So keep your portions small (around 3½ ounces or the size of your palm is the right amount for a meal), and alternate red meat with other protein sources.

**Lean poultry** Like red meat, the lean cuts supply more protein and other important minerals while limiting saturated fat intake—skinless breast and thigh fillets are the best choices.

**Fish and seafood** In addition to protein, these are a good source of zinc, iodine, vitamin B$_{12}$ and omega-3 fats. Fish with low mercury levels and high in omega-3 fats include mackerel, Atlantic salmon, canned salmon and canned tuna in oil, herring and sardines.

**Eggs** are a good source of protein, iron, zinc and vitamin B$_{12}$, and the omega-3 variety can also supply these important fats if you don't eat fish or seafood. However, eating too many eggs before or during pregnancy may increase the risk of gestational diabetes, so limit your intake to fewer than one per day.

**Tofu and tempeh** are good sources of protein for vegetarians or for anyone wanting a meat-free meal. They are rich in protein and are a good source of iron and zinc, while being low in saturated fat and cholesterol free.

**Legumes (including lentils, chickpeas and dried or canned beans)** These are versatile and economical protein sources that can be used in a range of dishes for both meat eaters and vegetarians. If your budget means that buying lean cuts of meat is a stretch, then swapping half the quantity of meat you use for legumes can provide both nutritional and cost benefits. They are a particularly important protein source for vegetarians.

**Quorn™** Also known as mycoprotein, this is a vegetarian protein source which can be used in place of meat in a variety of dishes—you can buy Quorn™ products from the supermarket freezer.

**Nuts and seeds** make a great protein-rich snack or addition to a meal, and also supply a range of other important vitamins and minerals.

**Whole grains** contain more protein as well as other vitamins and minerals, compared to their processed counterparts. Quinoa and bulgur are particularly high in protein.

**Dairy and soy products** Milk, yogurt, cheese and soy milk and soy yogurt all supply protein as well as calcium, zinc and vitamin $B_{12}$ (in dairy products and fortified soy products only). Other milk alternatives such as rice and oat milk contain much less protein.

## FREQUENTLY ASKED QUESTIONS

### "What if I am vegetarian or vegan?"

A well-planned vegetarian diet can provide all your nutritional requirements, including during pregnancy. Most of us eat more protein than we need and as long as you are eating enough food to provide your energy needs, it is quite easy to get enough protein in your diet. The key is to choose the protein foods that will also provide other important vitamins and minerals that can be more difficult to obtain in a vegetarian or vegan diet, such as iron, zinc, calcium and vitamin $B_{12}$. These include legumes (iron and zinc), tofu (iron, zinc and calcium), nuts and seeds (iron, zinc and calcium), fortified soy milk (calcium and vitamin $B_{12}$ if these are added), and, for those who eat them, dairy products (zinc, calcium and vitamin $B_{12}$) and eggs (iron, zinc and vitamin $B_{12}$). Whole grains are also a good source of protein for vegetarians, particularly quinoa and bulgur. While it was once thought that vegetarians needed to combine different protein foods at each meal, we now know this isn't necessary as long as you eat a variety of different protein foods throughout the day and from day to day.

## PROTEIN FOODS TO AVOID OR LIMIT IN PREGNANCY

**Fatty and processed meats** As well as being much lower in nutrient density, many of these are a food-safety risk, so should be avoided once pregnant. Processed meats have also been linked with

## STEP 4

# Keep your protein lean

an increased risk of type 2 diabetes, heart disease and cancer, so are something we should all limit, pregnant or not.

**Raw or undercooked meat, poultry or seafood.**

**Fish that are higher in mercury** including shark, swordfish, king mackerel, tilefish and bigeye or ahi (yellowfin) tuna.

**Raw or undercooked eggs** Eggs need to be thoroughly cooked when you are pregnant to reduce the risk of salmonella poisoning, so have them hard-boiled, scrambled or in an omelet.

## FREQUENTLY ASKED QUESTIONS

**"What if I am lactose intolerant?"**

Lactose intolerance means that you have low levels of the enzyme called lactase, which is needed to break down lactose (the natural sugar in milk) and allow it to be absorbed. Without adequate lactase, drinking too much milk or other milk products can cause symptoms of pain, bloating, gas and diarrhea. However, being lactose intolerant doesn't mean completely giving up dairy food. While milk, yogurt and custard are high in lactose, ice cream and soft cheeses (such as cottage) contain only moderate amounts of lactose, and hard cheeses have little to no lactose. Some people can still tolerate a moderate amount of milk and yogurt without developing symptoms, and yogurt is often better tolerated, as it contains good bacteria that help to digest the lactose. Lactose-free milks and yogurts (which are still made from dairy milk, and have the lactose already broken down) are also available. There is also a wide variety of dairy-milk substitutes to choose from, including soy, rice, almond or oat milk, but it is important to choose those that are fortified with calcium to ensure you still meet your calcium needs. Other good sources of calcium include canned fish with soft edible bones (such as salmon and sardines), calcium-set tofu, unhulled tahini, almonds, dried figs and some green leafy vegetables such as kale, collard greens and Chinese broccoli (gai lan).

**STEP**

# 5 Be choosy about fats

Having some fat in the diet is important to provide the body with essential fatty acids and to help with the absorption of fat-soluble vitamins; this is particularly important during pregnancy when the need for these fats is higher. But eating too much fat can be a problem, especially when it is the wrong type of fat.

## THE FACTS ABOUT FAT

The fats in our diet can be divided into three main types: saturated, monounsaturated and polyunsaturated. These can be further subdivided as shown in the diagram below.

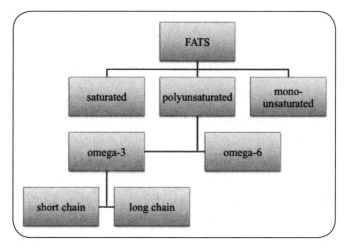

Foods that contain a high proportion of saturated fatty acids are solid at room temperature. These are commonly known as saturated fats and are found in animal foods and palm and coconut oils. Saturated fats are also found in processed foods that contain hydrogenated vegetable oil. All other plant fats— including those found in nuts, seeds, avocado and olives and most vegetable, nut and seed oils—are high in either polyunsaturated or monounsaturated fats. Saturated and monounsaturated fats are not

# 5 Be choosy about fats

necessary in the diet as they can be made in the body; however, mono-unsaturated fats have many other health benefits.

Polyunsaturated fats can be divided into omega-6 and omega-3 fatty acids, and omega-3 fats can be further divided into short-chain omega-3 fatty acids (from plants) and long-chain omega-3 fatty acids (from fish and seafood). Some types of polyunsaturated fats are what we call essential fatty acids. These are fats that are required for normal growth and development but cannot be made by our bodies, so we need to obtain them in our diets.

There are two essential fatty acids that we need: LA (linoleic acid) and ALA (alpha-linolenic acid). After digestion, LA and ALA are acted on by enzymes and converted to important fats (known as AA, EPA and DHA) that are used to regulate metabolism by acting as signals and altering cell membranes. Essential fatty acids are also needed for brain and eye development, so are particularly important in pregnancy, and can help in reducing inflammation and protecting against heart disease.

Research suggests that DHA and AA are both necessary for optimal development of the brain and eye. Newborns appear to have a limited ability to form AA and DHA, so your own intake of these important fats can improve your baby's stores before he or she is born. Most of the stores of these fatty acids are accumulated during the last trimester in pregnancy. DHA is also supplied by breast milk, but the amount varies depending on your intake. This means you should aim to get enough of these fats both during pregnancy and breastfeeding.

## THE FATS TO CHOOSE

Monounsaturated and polyunsaturated fats tend to lower levels of "bad" cholesterol, and monounsaturated fats can also increase "good" cholesterol, making them the best choices.

**Monounsaturated fats** are found in olives and olive oil, peanuts and peanut oil, avocados and avocado oil, macadamia nuts and macadamia oil and canola oil.

**Polyunsaturated fats** are found in sunflower, safflower and soybean oils, margarines made from these oils and many nuts and seeds.

**Omega-3 fats** are essential polyunsaturated fats that are found in fish, seafood, walnuts, flaxseeds and soybeans. These are particularly important in pregnancy as they are needed for your baby's eye and brain development.

## FATS TO AVOID

Saturated and trans fats tend to increase levels of bad cholesterol, and trans fats also reduce levels of good cholesterol, making them a particularly undesirable choice.

**Saturated fats** are found mainly in foods such as fatty meat and full-fat dairy products as well as in palm and coconut oils, which are commonly used in processed foods such as cookies, pastries and takeout.

**Trans fats** are found in products containing hydrogenated oils, such as cookies, cakes and fried takeout foods. Small amounts are present naturally in meat and dairy products. Some margarines contain trans fats.

## WAYS TO OPTIMIZE YOUR FAT INTAKE

» Choose only lean cuts of meat and skinless poultry, and include a few fish (or soy-based substitutes if you are vegetarian) meals per week.

» Choose low-fat dairy products, or try soy products instead.

» Use monounsaturated and polyunsaturated vegetable oils for cooking.

» Try flaxseed oil for salad dressings, particularly if you don't eat fish.

» Replace butter and mayonnaise with avocado, hummus, tahini or nut spreads (for example, almond butter).

# 5 STEP

## Be choosy about fats

» Avoid fried takeout foods and creamy sauces.

» Replace savory snacks like potato chips and corn chips with unsalted nuts and seeds.

» Make cookies, cakes, pastries and chocolate "indulgence" foods.

## FREQUENTLY ASKED QUESTIONS

### "How do I get enough omega-3 if I don't eat fish?"

While fish and seafood are the main sources of omega-3 in our diet, there are some other foods that contain these important fats. These include flaxseeds, flaxseed oil, canola oil, walnuts and soy products. You can include these in your diet by adding crushed flaxseeds to your cereal, using flaxseed oil in salad dressing (it can't be heated), snacking on a handful of walnuts or tossing some soybeans or tofu in a stir-fry. You could also choose omega-3 eggs (the hens are fed naturally occurring sources of omega-3, such as flaxseeds), and some breads, yogurts, milks, soy milks and fruit juices now have added omega-3. Fish oil supplements or vegetarian DHA supplements (from algae) can also be used, and many prenatal vitamins and mineral supplements now contain fish oil.

### "Is it safe to eat nuts during pregnancy?"

While some women are advised to avoid eating nuts during pregnancy and breastfeeding to reduce the risk of their baby developing allergies, there is actually no good evidence to suggest that this helps. In fact, the American Academy of Pediatrics (AAP), after reviewing the evidence regarding nutrition during pregnancy and breastfeeding and the development of allergies, says that there is no evidence to show that what a woman eats while pregnant or breastfeeding affects the chance of their child developing an allergy.

**"What is the best oil to cook with?"**

Different oils suit different types of cooking, cuisines and foods, and they can have different effects in terms of our health. Olive oil is one of the best choices, with a significant amount of research supporting its health benefits. The extra virgin variety comes from the first pressing of the olives (rather than being chemically extracted) and is darker in color with a stronger flavor, retaining more antioxidants than "light" olive oil. This is probably the best choice and is particularly suited to salad dressings, marinades and sautéing or panfrying. Light olive oil has a higher smoke point, so is better for use in stir-fries that require a higher temperature.

Canola, rice bran, avocado, peanut and macadamia oils also have a higher smoke point, making them good for stir-frying. Flaxseed oil and walnut oil make tasty salad dressings, providing healthy omega-3 fats, but they can't be heated, so shouldn't be used in cooking. Avoid "blended" vegetable oils, which are likely to contain some oils higher in saturated fat (like palm and coconut oils). Instead, always look for oils labeled "monounsaturated" and "polyunsaturated." Also check to make sure they don't contain any trans fats (which will be listed on the nutrition label).

## 6 STEP

# Be smart about carbs

While they seem to have got a bad name in recent years, carbohydrates are the main energy source for our muscles during vigorous exercise and the primary fuel for our brain. They should make up about half (40–60 percent) of our daily energy needs, particularly during pregnancy. Of course there are plenty of carbs that none of us need to be eating (such as cakes, pastries, cookies, highly processed cereals and crackers and white bread), but this doesn't mean all carbs are evil. In fact, there are plenty of carbs we should all be eating more of.

## THE LOW-CARB STORY

If you have been trying to lose weight, you may have tried or considered a low-carb/high-protein diet. Now that you are pregnant, or trying to conceive, you should think again.

While there is some research to suggest that diets higher in protein may have benefits for short-term weight loss, evidence for their long-term benefits is not as convincing. And there are many concerns about the potential long-term health implications of this type of eating plan—one that restricts whole grains, fruits and starchy vegetables. Not only are these foods important for the prevention of heart disease, diabetes and cancer, but high-protein diets and supplements have been linked with smaller babies with a high risk of illness at birth. Numerous studies have now linked high intakes of meat, particularly processed meats, with a greater chance of developing these diseases. More specifically, one study found that higher intake of red meat before pregnancy may increase the risk of gestational diabetes, while two studies found that women who ate one or more eggs each day may be more likely to develop the condition. Considering that it is difficult to follow a low-carb/high-protein diet without eating more eggs and red meat and that whole grains, fruit and vegetables are important contributors to nutrient intakes prior to and during pregnancy, this type of eating plan is not recommended once you are ready to conceive.

## FREQUENTLY ASKED QUESTIONS

**"I'm confused: What is the difference between whole grain and low GI?"**

Whole grain foods, including breads, cereals, brown rice, barley and oats have many health benefits—they are high in fiber and rich in important vitamins and minerals. But just because a food is labeled "whole grain" doesn't necessarily mean it has a low glycemic index.

**Whole grain foods** are those that contain all the components of the grain (the inner, middle and outside layers), but the grains may be intact, cracked, cooked, flaked, puffed, or milled, and it is this processing of the grain that can alter both the micronutrient content and the GI of the food. For example, whole wheat and whole grain breads are both considered to be whole grain foods, as they contain the entire grain, but in some breads, these grains are still intact, giving it a low GI, while in whole wheat bread, the grains have been milled to a fine texture, resulting in the bread having a high GI. Some breakfast cereals labeled whole grain have a high GI and have not been enriched, and they make poor carb choices.

For optimum health benefits, choose whole grain foods that also have a low GI. This includes whole grain breads (rather than whole wheat), traditional oatmeal and muesli (rather than cereals that have been puffed and flaked) and grains like barley, cracked wheat and quinoa.

## WHOLE GRAINS—THE CARBS TO FOCUS ON

In general, whole grain breads and cereals are nutritionally superior to more processed grains and flours, with higher levels of fiber, vitamins, minerals and phytochemicals. More importantly, eating just two to three servings of whole grain foods each day can reduce the risk of developing chronic diseases, such as heart disease, stroke, diabetes and certain cancers, by 20–30 percent. Despite this, on average, we are eating only one and a half servings per day—around half that

# 6 Be smart about carbs

needed to gain optimal health benefits. And if you are avoiding grains because of their higher carb intake, reconsider: Eating more whole grains has also been associated with a lower risk of being overweight and a reduced risk of weight gain.

## SLOW CARBS, NOT LOW-CARB

As we have said throughout this book, when it comes to carbs, your focus should be choosing the right carbs rather than cutting them out of your eating plan. Low GI carbs, the carbs that are more slowly digested and absorbed, not only provide more sustained energy and keep you fuller for longer, but can help to control blood glucose levels. If you have gestational diabetes, eating low GI meals will help to keep your post-meal blood glucose levels in the target range and may reduce the need for insulin.

Low GI carbs include some varieties of whole grain bread (look out for the low GI symbol), rolled oats, barley, legumes, quinoa, cracked wheat, pasta, corn, most fruits, dairy products, such as milk and yogurt, and soy milk.

## SUBSTITUTING LOW GI FOR HIGH GI FOODS

| HIGH GI FOOD | LOW GI ALTERNATIVE |
|---|---|
| Bread—white or whole wheat | Whole-grain bread and English muffins, sourdough and pumpernickel |
| Processed breakfast cereals | Choose unrefined cereals such as rolled oats or muesli, or a low GI processed cereal like All-Bran®. |
| Cookies or crackers | Pick cookies made with whole grains, oats and dried fruit. |
| Cakes and muffins | Make them with fruit, oats and whole grains. |

| HIGH GI FOOD | LOW GI ALTERNATIVE |
| --- | --- |
| Potato | Replace with red or baby new potatoes, sweet potatoes and corn. Make mashed potatoes with half cannellini beans. |
| Rice | Try longer grain varieties such as basmati or Uncle Ben's Converted Rice, or try pearled barley, quinoa, cracked wheat or noodles instead |

## QUALITY IS THE KEY

When it comes to carbs, the key is to choose quality: nutrient-dense, fiber-rich, low GI carbs that provide plenty of nutrition along with fiber to fill you up. Some good low GI swaps include:

» Choosing dense whole grain breads that have been certified low GI rather than white or whole wheat/brown breads

» Going for traditional thick-cut rolled oats rather than the instant or quick-cooking varieties

» Trying muesli rather than highly processed puffed and flaked cereals

» Looking for cereals that carry the low GI symbol, meaning that they have been officially tested and meet certain nutrition criteria—including All-Bran® and Special K®

» Using alternative whole grains such as barley, quinoa and cracked wheat in place of the standard rice, pasta and potatoes

» Switching from regular pasta to whole grain or whole wheat varieties—while all types of pasta have a low GI, the whole wheat and whole grain varieties have added nutritional benefits and are more filling

» Building legumes into your meals regularly—they not only supply protein, iron and zinc, but are a great source of slowly digested carbs and fiber

» Snacking on fruit, yogurt, crisp vegetable strips, roasted chickpeas and unsalted nuts and seeds in place of more processed snack foods.

# 6 Be smart about carbs

## FREQUENTLY ASKED QUESTIONS

**"What if I can't eat gluten?"**

Choosing the right carbs (whole grains and those with a low GI) can be more difficult for anyone who needs to avoid gluten due to celiac disease or gluten intolerance. Gluten is the protein found in wheat, rye, barley and oats, so a gluten-free diet cuts out many whole grain foods—and unfortunately, most gluten-free alternatives, including gluten-free breads, cereals, crackers and pasta, have a high GI. The good news is that there are also a number of whole grains and low GI carbs that are naturally gluten-free. These include brown rice (look for low GI varieties such as basmati), quinoa, buckwheat and legumes. And while you will benefit from eating low GI foods at each meal and for snacks, this doesn't have to be at the exclusion of all other carbs. Some high GI foods such as potatoes, gluten-free pasta or rice can make a valuable nutritional contribution to your diet, and when eaten with lean protein foods or low GI carbs such as beans, chickpeas or lentils, the overall glycemic response to the meal will be reduced.

# Don't forget your fluids

Many of us put a lot of effort into changing the foods we eat, but forget to consider what we are drinking. Keeping hydrated is important, particularly during pregnancy and breastfeeding. The amount of fluid we need each day varies depending on our activity levels, how much we sweat and the foods we eat (which also provide some fluid), but on average, a woman who isn't pregnant needs around 71 ounces of fluid per day, and this increases to 78 ounces in pregnancy and 88 ounces while breastfeeding. Be guided by your thirst, but also make sure you remember to drink regularly throughout the day and carry water with you when out, as it is easy to forget or even ignore your thirst if you are busy and don't have easy access to a drink. It is particularly important to stay well hydrated when exercising during pregnancy, as this helps to reduce the risk of overheating.

While we all know that water is the best choice to quench our thirst, few of us only drink water. Here, we give an overview of what's hot and what's not when it comes to fluid intake and pregnancy.

**Tea** Both green tea and black tea are rich in antioxidants known as catechins, which may help to protect against heart disease and cancer. The evidence for heart disease suggests tea may help to keep the lining of our blood vessels healthy and possibly reduce blood fat levels. More recently, scientists have discovered a compound in tea called theanine, which gives tea the ability to both relax you and improve mental clarity and concentration. On its own, tea is also calorie free, so it won't contribute to weight gain, unlike latte and hot chocolate, unless you add a lot of sugar and full-fat milk. However, like coffee, tea still contains a significant amount of caffeine, so if you are pregnant, you should have no more than five cups per day (and less if you are consuming other sources of caffeine).

# 7

## Don't forget your fluids

**Coffee** Current research suggests that in moderation (a few cups a day), coffee is safe to drink and may even offer some health benefits. For example, the risk of developing type 2 diabetes is lower among regular coffee drinkers, and research suggests coffee *may* reduce the risk of gallstones, colon cancer and Parkinson's disease. Coffee has also been shown to improve exercise endurance, and can help you to stay alert. But it is not completely harmless—the caffeine in coffee (and tea) is a stimulant that can increase heart rate and blood pressure, and can interfere with sleep. Too much caffeine during pregnancy may increase the risk of miscarriage and premature birth, and needs to be limited to around two cups of instant coffee or one cup of brewed coffee per day (or less if you consume other sources of caffeine). Caffeine also passes through into breast milk and may lead to an unsettled baby. Drinking too much can also affect milk production and may increase the risk of mastitis. For this reason, the American Academy of Pediatrics (AAP) recommends having no more than 300 milligrams (or around three cups of coffee) per day while breastfeeding. Like juices and smoothies, coffees have also become supersized these days and, if made with full-fat milk, can contribute a lot of energy and saturated fat—for example, a Starbucks Grande Latte with regular milk provides almost 220 calories and 11 grams of fat, making it more of a meal than a snack.

**Herbal teas** Herbal teas are made from the roots, berries, flowers, seeds and leaves of a variety of plants rather than from actual tea leaves. Herbal teas don't contain caffeine, but they do contain alkaloids, and there is some concern about consuming these during pregnancy as there is a lack of research on the safety of many herbs during pregnancy. For this reason, the FDA recommends caution when consuming herbal teas. While most commercial brands of herbal teas are thought to be safe to drink in reasonable amounts, those made with large amounts of herbs and those made with herbs known to be toxic are not. It is best to check with your doctor or midwife about the safety of herbal teas you wish to drink. Concentrated herbal supplements and drops are not a good idea for you or your baby.

**Fruit juice** Freshly squeezed 100 percent fruit juices offer a number of nutritional benefits, giving them an advantage over other sweet drinks, such as soda and sweetened juice drinks. They are a source of vitamins and minerals, including vitamin C, beta-carotene, folate, vitamin K and potassium. They can be an option if you are struggling to reach your quota of fruit and vegetables and are useful if you are having trouble gaining weight or have a poor appetite. They are not a replacement for fruit, however, as many don't contain the fiber of the whole fruit. If you like fresh juices, it is also important to realize that, like premade salads and fruit salads, these could be a food-safety risk if the fruit isn't well washed. It is therefore best to make these yourself. If you are watching your weight, juices are a concentrated source of energy (the same as soft drinks) that can add up the calories fast. It can take three or four pieces of fruit (or more, depending on the size) to make a glass of fruit juice, and while it would be difficult to eat the fruit in one sitting, most people have no trouble drinking a glass of fruit juice in a few minutes. If you are watching your weight, drink water and eat the whole fruit instead.

**Milk and soy milk** Whole milk is a good source of protein, calcium, zinc and vitamin $B_{12}$, but is high in saturated fat. Soy milk generally has a protein and fat content similar to dairy milk, but contains polyunsaturated rather than saturated fats. While soy milk doesn't naturally contain calcium or vitamin $B_{12}$, these are added to many brands (calcium more commonly than vitamin $B_{12}$), so the fortified varieties are the best choice to ensure you get enough of these nutrients. If you are watching your weight, it is a good idea to choose low-fat or skim/fat-free varieties, whether you have dairy or soy milk. If you choose other dairy alternatives such as rice, oat or almond milk, look for calcium-fortified varieties as these are

# Don't forget your fluids

all naturally low in calcium and also have a lower protein content than dairy or soy milk. If you don't like your milk plain, try adding a teaspoon of chocolate syrup, a few drops of vanilla or a sprinkle of cinnamon to warm milk. These are better options than buying flavored milks, which usually contain large amounts of added sugar.

**Smoothies and milkshakes** Smoothies and milkshakes made from low-fat dairy or soy products and fruit can make a satisfying healthy snack or light breakfast, and can be a great way to build fruit and calcium-rich foods into the diet. But they shouldn't be considered a drink to quench your thirst along with a meal—they are really a meal or a snack on their own. Despite sounding healthy, depending on the size, smoothies can be very high in fat and energy; for example, a 20-ounce Smoothie King Acai Adventure smoothie has 5 grams of fat and 456 calories—for a 155-pound female trying to limit weight gain, this is around one quarter of your daily energy needs. Like fresh juices, these also pose a food-safety risk in pregnancy—both soft-serve ice cream or yogurt and fruit that hasn't been washed well can contain *Listeria* bacteria. If you feel like a smoothie, it is best to make your own at home.

**Flavored ("vitamin") waters** While their labels promote a variety of health benefits, in reality, these are just water with some added sugar, flavors and selected vitamins or minerals. Most have around 5 to 7 percent added sugar, which is about half that of a soft drink, but their large size (most come in 16.9-ounce bottles) means that you will be consuming at least 25 grams (around six teaspoons) of sugar with each bottle. While they may appear to be a healthier option than other sweet drinks, you are better sticking to water and getting your vitamins from fresh fruit and vegetables, without the added sugar, colors and flavors.

**Alcohol** As discussed earlier in the book, avoiding alcohol altogether while pregnant or breastfeeding is known to be the safest option. And since you don't know you are pregnant in the early stages, it is best to avoid or limit alcohol once you are trying to conceive. It is particularly important to avoid binge drinking. If you continue to drink while trying to conceive, then limit your intake to no more than seven drinks per week and no more than two drinks on any one day. If you choose to drink while breastfeeding, limit your intake to no more than one or two drinks, and try to time your drink so that you minimize the alcohol in your breast milk—you can do this by having at least two hours between drinking and breastfeeding.

Tips for a healthy fluid intake:

» Water is the best thirst-quencher, contains no calories and is free—this should be your first choice for fluid. Make up a jug with slices of lemon or lime and keep in the fridge, or add a slice to a cup of hot water.

» Replace soft drinks and alcohol with plain seltzer or mineral water with a squeeze of lemon or lime.

» If you like fruit juice, have a small glass or dilute it with water or seltzer.

» When having smoothies, milkshakes or flavored milks, make sure you choose skim or low-fat milk or soy milk, and low-fat yogurt or ice cream, and go for smaller serving sizes.

» Avoid fresh fruit and vegetable juices (unless homemade) as these could be a food-safety risk.

» Don't leave home without a water bottle!

» Always have a pitcher of water on the dinner table at night.

» If your water at home or work doesn't taste great, invest in a water filter.

» If you are a big coffee drinker, you could replace some with tea (but still limit your total intake of caffeine), or try a hot milk drink or warm soy milk instead.

# Avoid harm

So far, we have focused on what you should eat, but there are also some foods and fluids that are best avoided or limited when you are pregnant, breastfeeding or trying to conceive. We have discussed these earlier in the book, but here is a quick overview of what to look out for.

## FOODS TO AVOID OR LIMIT

| TRYING TO CONCEIVE | PREGNANCY | BREASTFEEDING |
|---|---|---|
| Avoid or limit alcohol to no more than 7 drinks per week and no more than 2 drinks per day. Avoid binge drinking at all costs. | Avoid alcohol—there is no safe level, but binge drinking presents the highest risk. | Avoid alcohol, or consider the timing in relation to feeding. |
| Cut down on caffeine to less than 2–3 cups of coffee per day. | Avoid or limit caffeine (no more than 200mg/day—see page 52. | Avoid or limit caffeine, and consider timing in relation to breastfeeding. |
| Quit smoking with medical and family support. | Don't smoke. | Don't smoke. |
| Limit intake of high-mercury fish (shark, swordfish, king mackerel, tilefish and bigeye or ahi/yellowfin tuna). | Avoid high-mercury fish (shark, swordfish, king mackerel, tilefish and bigeye or ahi/yellowfin tuna). | Avoid or limit high-mercury fish (shark, swordfish, king mackerel, tilefish and bigeye or ahi/yellowfin tuna). |
| Avoid supplements containing high doses of vitamin A and skin products containing retinoids. | Avoid supplements containing high doses of vitamin A and skin products containing retinoids. | Avoid supplements containing high doses of vitamin A and skin products containing retinoids. |

| TRYING TO CONCEIVE | PREGNANCY | BREASTFEEDING |
|---|---|---|
| If you take any vitamin, mineral or herbal supplements, check that these are safe during pregnancy, and consider changing to a prenatal vitamin or folate. | Avoid any vitamin, mineral or herbal supplements, unless you have checked they are safe during pregnancy. A prenatal vitamin is usually the best choice. | Avoid any vitamin, mineral or herbal supplements, unless you have checked they are safe while breastfeeding. A prenatal vitamin is usually the best choice. |
| Be aware of high-risk foods to avoid exposure to *Listeria, Salmonella and Toxoplasma gondii*. | Avoid foods that may contain *Listeria* (including soft cheeses, cold meats and chicken, raw seafood, pâté, unpasteurized dairy products, pre-prepared salads and fruit salads, and soft-serve ice cream), *Salmonella* (raw/ undercooked eggs and bean sprouts) or *Toxoplasma gondii* (raw or undercooked meats). Practice good food hygiene.<br><br>Wash hands well after contact with animals, wear gloves when gardening and avoid handling kitty litter. | Continue to practice good food hygiene for you and your baby. |

# Chapter 11

# Putting it all together

| | |
|---|---|
| **1** Scrutinize your current food intake and work out what to change— use our "swap this for that" approach | **2** Plan your meals and snacks for the week ahead |
| **3** Write a shopping list and stock your fridge and pantry | **4** Start each day with a nutritious low GI breakfast |
| **5** Pack a healthy lunch and snacks if you won't be at home | **6** Keep the plate model in mind when planning your meals (see pages 186–90) |
| **7** Prepare meals ahead for the nights you don't feel like cooking | **8** Try one or two new recipes each week |
| **9** Experiment with foods you don't usually eat, such as legumes, quinoa and barley | **10** Always keep food safety in mind |

We hope by now that you have a good idea of the foods to eat (and those to avoid) in pregnancy or while planning, and how to build low GI foods into your meals. But just to bring it all together and make it as easy as possible to plan your meals, this is an example of how it should look.

## BREAKFAST

This really is the most important meal of the day. Even if you are always in a rush in the mornings, it is well worth making five or ten minutes to eat this meal.

1. Choose high-fiber cereal based on oats or barley, or dense whole grain breads/toast.
2. Add some protein to keep you satisfied for longer—good choices include low-fat milk or yogurt, canned fish, eggs, low-fat hard cheese or cottage cheese and nuts or nut spreads.
3. Toss in some fruit or vegetables for a healthy dose of fiber, vitamins and antioxidants. Try berries with muesli and yogurt, stewed apples in oatmeal, grilled tomatoes and mushrooms with eggs or asparagus on toast plus an orange.

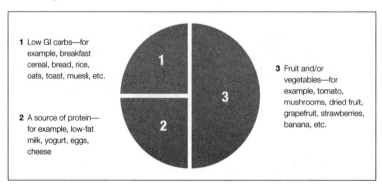

1 Low GI carbs—for example, breakfast cereal, bread, rice, oats, toast, muesli, etc.

2 A source of protein—for example, low-fat milk, yogurt, eggs, cheese

3 Fruit and/or vegetables—for example, tomato, mushrooms, dried fruit, grapefruit, strawberries, banana, etc.

Try these suggestions for a tasty, nutritious breakfast:

» Traditional oatmeal with soy milk and sliced banana
» Bircher muesli with yogurt and berries
» Low GI whole grain toast with natural peanut butter or almond spread
» Sardines and tomato on low GI whole grain toast

» Fruit salad with yogurt and a sprinkle of muesli (if toasted, make sure it is based on healthy fat)
» Toasted rye sourdough with grilled cheese and tomato
» Low-fat milk or soy milk berry smoothie with oats and chia seeds
» Scrambled eggs with grilled tomato and baby spinach on whole grain toast.

## LUNCH

Taking a break for a satisfying lunchtime meal is important for maintaining energy levels and concentration and preventing hunger and nausea. Whether you are eating at home, taking lunch with you or buying a meal out, there are plenty of healthy choices available.

1. Pick your low GI carbs: Try a whole grain bread or roll, Ryvita® or Kavli crispbreads, pasta or noodles, low GI rice, quinoa, barley, legumes or cracked wheat.
2. Add a good serving of vegetables or salad.
3. Finish with a small amount of lean protein: Good choices include canned fish, hard-boiled eggs, home-cooked meat or chicken, marinated tofu, hard cheese and legumes. Avoid processed/deli meats, smoked salmon and soft cheeses.

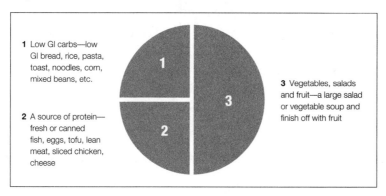

1 Low GI carbs—low GI bread, rice, pasta, toast, noodles, corn, mixed beans, etc.

2 A source of protein— fresh or canned fish, eggs, tofu, lean meat, sliced chicken, cheese

3 Vegetables, salads and fruit—a large salad or vegetable soup and finish off with fruit

The options are endless but here are a few ideas to get you started:
» Whole grain sandwich with canned tuna and salad
» Garden salad with chicken, avocado and croutons made from whole wheat bread cut into cubes and baked in the oven. Dress with a mixture of olive oil, vinegar, lemon juice and a teaspoon of honey.

» Vegetable frittata made with sweet potato, bell peppers, peas and corn
» Bowl of minestrone or lentil and vegetable soup
» Asparagus and bell pepper quiches: Use whole grain bread rolled out and pressed into muffin cups in place of piecrust.
» Ryvita® or Kavli crispbread with tuna, tomato and cucumber
» Tuna-pasta salad: Combine cold pasta spirals, canned tuna, snow peas and cherry tomatoes, and make a dressing from plain yogurt, lemon juice and fresh herbs.
» Mini-muffin pizzas using multigrain English muffins topped with tomato, red and green bell pepper slices, mushrooms and a sprinkle of grated mozzarella
» Roasted hot or cold vegetable salad (try bell peppers, zucchini, squash or sweet potato and eggplant brushed with olive oil and baked) with chickpeas, baby spinach leaves and a dash of balsamic vinegar.

## SNACKS

There is nothing wrong with eating between meals if you are hungry. And if you are pregnant, eating three small meals and two to three snacks can help ensure you are getting all the nutrients you and your baby need while also helping with nausea and heartburn. But most processed snack foods are high in fat, sugar or salt and are best left on the shelf. Try to choose nutrient-dense snack foods and avoid "empty calories." Look for those carrying the certified GI symbol.

Good choices include:
» A piece of fresh fruit
» A small handful of unsalted nuts and seeds or dried fruit and nuts
» A small bowl of berries with a dollop of plain yogurt
» Two or three Ryvita® or Kavli crispbreads with cottage cheese and tomato
» Tzatziki or hummus dip (look for low-fat and reduced-sodium varieties, or make your own) with raw carrot and celery
» Whole grain cinnamon raisin bagel with low-fat cream cheese (neufchâtel)
» A handful of roasted chickpeas
» A small container of low-fat yogurt

» Homemade "healthy" muffins made with whole wheat stone-ground flour, oats, oat bran, nuts, fresh or dried fruit and a healthy oil rather than butter—see our recipe section for ideas.

## DINNER

When you are tired after a long day, it can be hard to get motivated to cook. But putting a meal together at the end of the day doesn't have to take a lot of time and effort. The key is to keep your kitchen stocked with the right foods—use our shopping list to make sure you have everything you need.

1. Fill half of your plate with a variety of different non-starchy vegetables or salads—aim to make your plate as colorful as possible.

2. Fill another quarter of your plate with some low-fat protein—fish, seafood, lean meat, skinless poultry, eggs, tofu or legumes.

3. Fill the remaining quarter of your plate with low GI/high-fiber carbs—whole grain pasta or noodles, basmati rice, barley, quinoa, cracked wheat, corn, sweet potato or legumes.

4. For flavor, use fresh or dried herbs and spices, garlic, ginger, chili, lemon and lime juice, a small amount of honey, vinegar, olive oil, no-salt-added canned crushed tomatoes or tomato purée. Avoid most prepared sauces, as these are usually high in fat, sugar and/or salt.

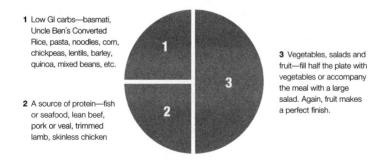

1 Low GI carbs—basmati, Uncle Ben's Converted Rice, pasta, noodles, corn, chickpeas, lentils, barley, quinoa, mixed beans, etc.

2 A source of protein—fish or seafood, lean beef, pork or veal, trimmed lamb, skinless chicken

3 Vegetables, salads and fruit—fill half the plate with vegetables or accompany the meal with a large salad. Again, fruit makes a perfect finish.

Here are just a few suggestions:

» Small grilled lean steak with cob of corn and garden salad
» Baked salmon fillet with homemade French fries (using new potatoes, sliced and brushed with olive oil) and steamed carrots, broccoli and beans
» Quinoa with roasted vegetables (such as bell peppers, eggplant, zucchini and squash) and chickpeas
» Tofu and vegetable stir-fry with Hokkien noodles
» Lean lamb kebabs with hummus and salad
» Barley risotto with mushrooms, bell peppers, spinach, peas and sliced skinless chicken breast
» Chicken and lentil curry with basmati rice and steamed greens
» Corn tortillas filled with a mixture of lean ground beef and kidney beans (cooked with onion, garlic, chili and canned crushed tomatoes) and chopped tomato, lettuce, cucumber and mashed avocado
» Lentil shepherd's pie using a mixture of lentils, vegetables and canned tomatoes for the filling and mashed potatoes and cannellini beans on top
» Chickpea and vegetable curry with a small serving of brown basmati rice
» A bowl of homemade minestrone or vegetable and lentil soup (great to make ahead of time and have frozen for a night when you don't feel like cooking)
» Homemade pizza using a whole grain wrap as the base and topped with tomato purée, roasted vegetables (for example, squash, eggplant, zucchini and bell peppers), avocado and a sprinkle of mozzarella and pine nuts.

# Chapter 12

# Stocking your pantry

Preparing and eating healthy meals starts with having the right ingredients. Having a well-stocked pantry means you can always have things on hand to put together a quick and healthy meal, saving you time, energy and money.

# GRAINS AND LEGUMES

These foods should feature regularly in your meals. They are the major contributors to healthy carbs in your diet. Go for whole grain varieties most of the time.

**Barley** adds flavor and fiber to soups and stews and can also be used as a tasty and nutritious alternative to rice in dishes like risotto and pilaf. It has the lowest GI of all grains at just 25, making it a particularly good choice. Store barley in an airtight glass container in a cool, dark, dry place or in the refrigerator during warmer weather.

**Barley bran** is another option and is usually available in the cereal section of supermarket or health-food stores.

**Bulgur (cracked wheat)** is most commonly used in making tabbouli salad. It has a GI value of 48. Bulgur will keep for six months stored in an airtight container in the refrigerator.

**Couscous** is a quick-cooking grain that can be used in salads or as a base for casseroles in place of rice or pasta. Couscous will keep well for a year stored in airtight bags or containers. Pearl couscous (larger grain) has a lower GI.

**Dried legumes** Legumes, or pulses, are low in fat, high in fiber, and are a good source of protein, low GI carbohydrates (most have GI values between 20 and 40), B vitamins, folate and minerals, including iron and zinc. They are economical, filling and versatile and are certainly not just for vegetarians, but something we should all be eating more of. People often don't know what to do with legumes, so try lentil-based curries, chickpeas added to stir-fries, cannellini bean mash or cranberry beans in your favorite winter casserole. Dried beans will keep for up to two years in an airtight container in a cool dry place.

**Dried noodles and pasta** While most types of pasta and noodles have a low GI, choose whole grain or whole wheat varieties for added fiber and nutrition. Store in an airtight container away from moisture. Dried noodles and pasta can be stored indefinitely and still be safe to eat, but for best quality, keep for no more than two years.

**Quinoa (pronounced keen-wah)** is a nutritious, quick-cooking grain, similar to couscous but wheat- and gluten-free, and high in protein, iron and fiber. It has a lower GI (53) than couscous and this, combined with its nutritional benefits, makes it a great alternative. It can be made into cereal or dessert, or used as a grain in meals in place of couscous or rice. Quinoa will keep for a year if stored in an airtight container in a cool, dark, dry place.

**Rice** Choose the lower GI basmati rice or Uncle Ben's Converted Rice, or brown rice for more fiber and iron. As most varieties of brown rice are higher GI, brown basmati is the best option, although it can be harder to find. White rice will keep for a year stored in a sealed container in a cool dry place. Brown rice should be kept in an airtight container in the refrigerator and will keep for six months.

**Rolled oats** are the perfect breakfast cereal, either cooked as oatmeal in winter or made into muesli in summer. They can also be used in baking muffins or cookies. Choose the whole or "traditional" oats rather than the instant or quick-cooking varieties, which have a higher GI. Keep oats in an airtight container and store in a cool dark place for up to three months, or in the refrigerator for up to six months.

# CANNED FOODS

Cans should be kept in a dry place to prevent rusting. Although they can technically be kept indefinitely, for optimum quality and nutrition, use within twelve months. Discard any cans that are swollen, badly dented and/or rusted. When available, choose no-salt-added or reduced-salt varieties.

**Canned beans** are a handy alternative when you don't have time to prepare the dried variety. Rinse and drain well, then use in similar ways to the dried variety. They don't need cooking, so can be used in salads or added toward the end of cooking to heat through. Any unused portion should be stored in an airtight container in the fridge and used within a few days, or can be frozen for use at another time.

**Canned tomatoes** should be a staple in every healthy pantry. They can be used in pasta dishes, soups, casseroles, and curries, and are a better alternative to prepared pasta sauces, which usually contain added salt and sugar. Choose the crushed variety, and add your own fresh or dried herbs and spices for the perfect tomato-based sauce.

**Canned tuna and salmon** are a great alternative to fresh fish, and are rich in healthy omega-3 fats (particularly salmon). They can be added to salads or sandwiches, made into patties or stirred into pasta for a quick healthy meal.

**Canned sardines** While less popular than tuna and salmon, sardines are the richest source of long-chain omega-3 fats, providing up to ten times more than canned tuna. They are also a good source of calcium (due to their small, edible bones) and rich in vitamin D and iodine. Best of all, sardines are a versatile, economical food and, being low on the food chain, they are likely to have lower levels of contaminants such as mercury, compared to other deep-sea fish. Serve them on toast for breakfast or lunch.

# OILS, VINEGARS, SAUCES AND CONDIMENTS

The right selection of cooking oils and flavors can help to make quick easy meals that are tasty while still being good for you. While prepared cooking sauces may be easy, most are high in fat, salt and/or sugar. Having a selection of good basic ingredients makes it easy to prepare your own tasty meals without the additives.

**Asian sauces** such as soy sauce, sweet chili sauce, Thai curry paste, hoisin sauce, oyster sauce, tandoori paste and miso are a great way to liven up simple meals, although they tend to be high in salt, so choose reduced-sodium varieties whenever available. Asian oils, vinegars and soy sauce can be kept at room temperature away from light and heat, while other sauces and pastes should generally be refrigerated after opening.

**Extra virgin olive oil** is great for use in salads and low-heat cooking (including stir-frying). For optimum flavor and to prevent oxidation, buy those that are sold in dark tinted bottles or metal containers. Store away from light and heat, and use within six months.

**Flaxseed oil** Made from flaxseeds, this oil is rich in plant omega-3 fats and a great option for vegetarians or non-fish eaters. It needs to be kept in a dark bottle in the fridge and can't be heated, but it makes a great salad dressing, providing a nutty flavor. It can also be added to smoothies.

**Olives** Store unopened jars of olives in a cool place for up to two years. After opening, keep in the refrigerator and use within two weeks.

**Sesame oil** is used in small amounts to add flavor to Asian meals such as stir-fries and salads. Like other oils, it should be stored away from light and heat and can be kept in the fridge.

**Stock** Fresh stock can be kept in a covered container in the refrigerator for three days, or frozen for six months (three months for fish stock). Liquid stock or bouillon cubes without MSG have a long shelf life, but should be kept in a cool dry place. Choose reduced-sodium varieties.

**Sun-dried tomatoes** Unopened jars of sun-dried tomatoes packed in oil will keep for a year without refrigeration. After opening, refrigerate and use within nine months.

**Tomato purée** can be used in a variety of meals, including pasta sauces and homemade pizzas. Once opened, store any leftovers in a container in the fridge for two to three days, or freeze in ice-cube trays for convenient future use. Choose no-salt-added varieties.

**Vegetable oils** Other good options for cooking include canola, peanut, rice bran, avocado and nut oils. Different oils can be used for different dishes depending on the flavor you are after—for example, peanut oil for Asian stir-fries or nut oils for salads. Canola and rice bran oils are good for higher temperature cooking or where you don't want flavor from the oil, such as in baking. Look for mono-unsaturated or polyunsaturated oils, and avoid blended vegetable oils that can contain palm oil (high in saturated fat).

**Vinegar** comes in a variety of flavors, including white wine, red wine, balsamic, malt and apple cider, all suited to different dishes. If stored in a cool dark place, unopened bottles of vinegar will keep indefinitely. Vinegar should be used within six months after opening, and kept in a cool dark place or in the refrigerator.

# HERBS AND SPICES

Keep a selection of basil, bay leaves, cayenne pepper, chili powder/flakes, cinnamon, cloves, cilantro, cumin, curry powder, ginger, nutmeg, oregano, paprika, pepper, rosemary, turmeric and thyme available. All herbs and spices should be kept in airtight containers in a cool, dark and dry place and used within one year. Fresh herbs can also be grown easily at home.

# DRIED FRUITS, NUTS AND SEEDS

Nuts and dried fruit are nature's perfect snack food, packed with nutrition and minus the added sugar, salt, fat and packaging of most processed snack foods. They can also be used in baking healthy muffins, cakes and cookies or added to cereals, and a sprinkle of nuts and seeds adds flavor to salads, pasta dishes, curries and stir-fries.

**Dried fruit** is great to have on hand for snacking, in casseroles or poached for dessert. Dried fruit stored in airtight containers in a cool dry place will keep well for six to twelve months. Choose naturally dried fruits where possible.

**Nuts** provide a nutritional package not found in any other one food. They are rich in healthy fats, a good source of plant protein and high in dietary fiber, while also being a good source of important vitamins and minerals, including iron, zinc and folate, and rich in antioxidants and phytochemicals. And despite their high fat content, research has shown that people who eat nuts regularly are less likely to be overweight. Nuts absorb odors, so keep in an airtight container in a cool, dark and dry place. They will last for four months if shelled and six months in the shell. To extend their shelf life, place them in the refrigerator where they will keep for nine months, or freeze for up to two years. Choose the raw, unsalted variety for maximum nutrition.

**Nut spreads** Natural nut spreads, or butters, are basically nuts ground to a coarse paste and include peanut, almond, and macadamia. These can be found in your supermarket or in health-food stores. By choosing these natural varieties, you avoid the extra fat, sugar and salt added to the more processed spreads.

**Seeds** are an often forgotten, but nutritionally packed, food. Like nuts, they are high in dietary fiber, are a rich source of healthy unsaturated fats and vitamin E, and provide a range of important minerals. The most commonly eaten seeds are sunflower and pumpkin seeds. Because these tend to be eaten in larger amounts than other seeds, they are a good source of protein, iron and zinc. Flaxseeds can be used whole or ground and added to cereal, breads and muffins. They are one of the richest plant sources of omega-3 fatty acids, which we know are important in pregnancy. Chia seeds come from the plant *Salvia hispanica*, native to Central and South America, and like flaxseeds, are a rich source of plant-based omega-3 fats and fiber. They look a bit like tiny sesame seeds and come in black or white, providing a variety of vitamins and minerals including iron, calcium, magnesium and potassium.

**Tahini** Made from ground sesame seeds, tahini is tasty spread on toast or sandwiches, drizzled over salads or roasted vegetables, or used in dips like hummus and baba ganoush. The unhulled variety is a particularly good source of calcium, important for those who don't eat dairy products.

# FROZEN FOODS

Keeping a few basics in the freezer can help for days when you don't have time to shop for fresh foods.

**Frozen berries** These are great for adding to plain yogurt as a snack, on top of cereal for breakfast or in a smoothie.

**Frozen vegetables** Keep a supply of frozen peas, corn, beans and stir-fry mix at the ready for healthy meals when you're short on time. Research has shown that these are equivalent to, or sometimes even better than fresh when it comes to nutrition, as they are usually flash-frozen as soon as they are picked. Frozen vegetables will keep for eight months at 0°F/18°C.

**Whole grain bread**, when frozen in airtight bags, will keep for three months, and can be used for toasting or toasted sandwiches.

**Whole grain English muffins** Freeze whole grain English muffins in airtight bags and use within three months. Choose the whole grain variety for an easy breakfast option, healthy snack, alternative pizza base or an easy lunch or dinner meal topped with scrambled eggs.

# FRESH FOODS

**Cheese** is a good source of protein, calcium and zinc, but can also be high in saturated fat, cholesterol and salt. Try reduced-fat and reduced-sodium versions of hard cheese and low-fat cream and cottage cheeses. Soft cheeses, including brie, camembert, ricotta and feta, should be avoided during pregnancy due to *Listeria* risk.

**Eggs** are an excellent source of protein, and a good source of iron, zinc, vitamin D and vitamin $B_{12}$. Omega-3 eggs are a good way to boost your intake of omega-3 fats if you don't eat fish or seafood. They are a quick and easy meal option, but as some studies have linked high intakes (more than seven per week) with an increased risk of gestational diabetes and type 2 diabetes, it is best to limit your intake and alternate with other protein sources. Eggs must be well-cooked in pregnancy due to the risk of *Salmonella*.

**Fish, particularly oily fish**, are the best dietary source of long-chain omega-3 fatty acids, which are important during pregnancy and breastfeeding. Varieties of fish that contain the highest amounts of omega-3 fats include Atlantic salmon, rainbow trout, blue mackerel, canned sardines, canned salmon and some varieties of canned tuna. Fish that are higher in mercury include shark, swordfish, king mackerel, tilefish and bigeye or ahi (yellowfin) tuna—these varieties should be limited or avoided during pregnancy, breastfeeding and for young children.

**Fruit and vegetables** should form a major part of any healthy eating plan. They are rich sources of vitamins, minerals, antioxidants and phytochemicals, all of which are important for good health and can help to protect against diseases such as cancer and heart disease. They are also high in fiber, helping to fill you up, and, apart from avocado and olives (which contain healthy monounsaturated fats), fruits and vegetables contain little fat. You should aim to eat at least five servings of vegetables and salads and two servings of fruit each day. When choosing fruits and vegetables, variety is the key—aim to make your plate as colorful as possible. It is important that fruit and vegetables are well washed when you are pregnant, to avoid the risk of *Listeria*, particularly if you are eating them raw. Avoid bean sprouts and premade salads or fruit salads.

**Meat and poultry** are good sources of protein, iron, zinc and vitamin $B_{12}$. Choose lean cuts of meat and skinless poultry to avoid excess saturated fat and cholesterol and to maximize nutrition. Where cost is an issue, choose small amounts of lean meat or poultry, and use in dishes such as stir-fries, curries, casseroles and stews, along with legumes and lots of vegetables.

**Milk or alternatives** Regular dairy milk is a good source of protein, calcium, zinc and vitamin B$_{12}$. Choose reduced-fat or skim varieties to reduce your intake of saturated fat and energy, particularly if you are watching your weight. If you use milk alternatives such as soy, rice, almond, or oat milk, choose those fortified with calcium to ensure you are still getting an adequate intake of this important mineral. Oat and rice milk are lower in protein and are not recommended for infants or children under five years of age.

**Tofu**, also known as bean curd, is a soybean product made by curdling fresh soy milk. Usually sold in rectangular blocks, tofu is an off-white color and has a neutral taste, absorbing the flavors of surrounding ingredients. Tofu is a great source of protein and iron (particularly for vegetarians), a good source of calcium and low in saturated fat. There are two main kinds of tofu. Silken tofu has a smoother texture and is best suited for salad dressings, sauces and desserts, while firm and hard tofu are best for baking, stir-frying and grilling. Once opened, tofu should be rinsed well and kept covered with water in a sealed container in the refrigerator. Change the water daily to keep the tofu fresh, and use within one week.

**Yogurt** is made from milk that is fermented with live bacteria cultures. It is high in protein and one of the best dietary sources of calcium, as well as supplying valuable B-group vitamins. Extra cultures are often added, which can help restore the body's natural gut flora and be beneficial to digestive health. There is also increasing evidence that these bacteria can help to improve our immune system. Plain yogurt is the best choice, as it comes without the added sugar and calories of flavored varieties and is more versatile—use it in salad dressings, dips, curries and soups, or team it with fruit or nuts for a healthy snack or dessert.

## SHOPPING FOR LOW GI FOODS

GI values are the key to lowering the GI of your diet. Unfortunately, not every food has been tested for its GI, and some manufacturers make low GI claims that are not based on proper testing. Many people assume that all whole grain foods are slowly digested and absorbed—which is far from true. However, you can look up reliable GI values of a large number of carbohydrate-containing foods by consulting these two sources of information:

» The free online searchable database at glycemicindex.com. This database is maintained by the University of Sydney and is regularly updated with new values as they come to hand. The website also gives you access to a free monthly electronic newsletter called *GI News* (ginewsblogspot.com).

» The *Shopper's Guide* is a pocket-size book published annually under the series title The Low GI Shopper's Guide to GI Values. This inexpensive, easy-to-use guide helps you compare your favorite foods and preferred brands so you can make substitutions that really matter.

# HOW DO I KNOW IT'S TRULY A LOW GI FOOD?

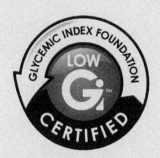

**Look for the Low GI Symbol**

Low and medium GI foods can carry the symbol, provided they meet the nutrient criteria. This means they have a GI of 69 or lower. (Low GI foods are those with a GI value of 55 or lower.)

The GI symbol makes healthy shopping easier. When you see this logo on a product, it means it's been assessed by the experts, and ticked all the boxes. It's your guarantee that the GI value stated near the nutrition information table is accurate. Foods that carry the certified GI symbol have been judged against a range of nutrient criteria, so you can be sure that the food is a healthy nutritional choice within its food group (for example, dairy or bread). The program is administered by the Glycemic Index Foundation, a nonprofit organization established by the University of Sydney, Diabetes Australia and the Juvenile Diabetes Research Foundation, Australia. Manufacturers pay the GI Foundation a license fee to use the certified symbol on their products, and the income is channeled back into education and research. You can find out more at gisymbol.com.

# Chapter 13

# Top pregnancy super foods

So far, we have discussed the most important nutrients to include in your diet for pregnancy and conception, but in this chapter we outline exactly how much of each of these key nutrients you need when you are trying to conceive, while you are pregnant and when you are breastfeeding. We also show you the best food sources of these nutrients and how much they supply, so you can make sure you are getting enough. Of course, individual needs can vary, so consider getting some tailored nutrition advice from a registered dietitian (RD), particularly if you have any other health problems that may impact your nutritional needs.

# IMPORTANT NUTRIENT SUMMARY TABLE

| NUTRIENT | HOW MUCH YOU NEED BEFORE CONCEPTION (DAILY INTAKE)* | HOW MUCH YOU NEED WHEN PREGNANT (DAILY INTAKE)* | HOW MUCH YOU NEED WHEN BREASTFEEDING (DAILY INTAKE)* | WHERE YOU CAN FIND IT |
|---|---|---|---|---|
| Folate | 400 mcg | 600 mcg | 500 mcg | Green leafy vegetables, legumes, avocado, oranges, nuts, wheat germ, fortified breads and cereals |
| Iron | 18 mg | 27 mg | 9 mg | Lean red meat, legumes, tofu, whole grains, green leafy vegetables, dried fruits, nuts |
| Calcium | 1,000 mg | 1,000 mg | 1,000 mg | Milk, yogurt, cheese, fortified soy milk, firm tofu, soy yogurt, unhulled tahini, almonds, dried figs, Asian greens, kale |
| Omega-3 fats | 500 mg | 500 mg | 650 mg | ALA: flaxseeds, walnuts, chia seeds, flaxseed oil<br><br>EPA/DHA: Oily fish, eggs |
| Iodine | 150 mcg | 220 mcg | 290 mcg | Seafood, sea vegetables, iodized salt, fortified bread, dairy products, eggs, some vegetables |
| Vitamin D | 15 mcg | 15 mcg | 15 mcg | Oily fish, milk, eggs, butter, margarines, fortified milks and soy milks. Exposure to safe levels of sunlight. |

* Values are for women aged 19–50 years; for women under 19 years, the intake of some nutrients is increased.

# FOLATE SUPER FOODS

| FOOD | FOLATE CONTENT (MICROGRAMS, MCG) |
|---|---|
| Peanuts (raw), 1½ tablespoons (40 g) | 96 |
| Spinach, ½ cup boiled | 85 |
| Baked beans, ½ cup canned | 75 |
| Avocado, ½ medium | 71 |
| Chickpeas, ½ cup cooked | 63 |
| Orange, 1 medium | 56 |
| Whole grain bread, 1 slice* | 54 |
| Asparagus, 4 spears, cooked | 38 |
| Wheat germ, 2 tablespoons | 33 |
| Brussels sprouts, 4 medium | 32 |
| Red kidney beans, ½ cup cooked | 32 |
| Broccoli, ½ cup cooked | 30 |
| Lentils, ½ cup cooked | 20 |
| Cabbage, ½ cup cooked | 8 |

\* Excluding organic breads, which don't have added folate

# IRON SUPER FOODS

| FOOD | IRON CONTENT (MG) |
|---|---|
| Quinoa, ¼ cup uncooked | 3.9 |
| Muesli, ½ cup (untoasted) | 3.5 |
| Tofu, firm, 3½ ounces | 2.9 |
| Lean fillet steak, 3½ ounces (100 g) | 2.2 |
| Lentils, ½ cup cooked | 2.0 |
| Chickpeas, ½ cup cooked | 1.8 |
| Lamb chop, trimmed, 3½ ounces (100 g) | 1.5 |
| Almonds, 2 tablespoons (30 g) | 1.2 |
| Atlantic salmon fillet, 3½ ounces (100 g) | 1.1 |
| Tuna, canned, 3½ ounces (100 g) | 1.1 |
| Egg, 1 hard-boiled | 0.8 |
| Whole grain bread, 1 slice | 0.6 |
| Boneless pork chop, 3½ ounces (100 g) | 0.6 |
| Chicken breast, 3½ ounces (100 g) | 0.4 |

# CALCIUM SUPER FOODS

| FOOD | CALCIUM CONTENT (MG) |
| --- | --- |
| Sardines, canned, 3½ ounces (100 g) | 430 |
| Yogurt, plain, 6-ounce container (170 g) | 200–300 |
| Milk, low-fat, 1 cup | 300 |
| Milk, regular, 1 cup | 246 |
| Fortified soy beverage, 1 cup | 250–300 |
| Cheese, 25 percent reduced fat, 1½ slices | 320 |
| Firm tofu, 3½ ounces (100 g) | 320 |
| Bok choy, 1 cup cooked | 280 |
| Salmon, pink, canned, 3½ ounces (100 g) | 200 |
| Dried figs, 4 | 150 |
| Unhulled tahini, 1 tablespoon | 83 |
| Soy beverage, unfortified, 1 cup | 61 |
| Almonds, 2 tablespoons | 75 |
| Broccoli, 1 cup cooked | 52 |
| Kale, 1 cup cooked | 45 |

# OMEGA-3 FATS SUPER FOODS

| FOOD | OMEGA-3 CONTENT (MG) |
| --- | --- |
| Flaxseed oil, 1 tablespoon | 9,830* |
| Flaxseeds, 1 tablespoon | 2,765* |
| Atlantic salmon, 3½ ounces (100 g) | 2,050 |
| Chia seeds, 1 tablespoon | 1,930* |
| Walnuts, 2 tablespoons | 1,885* |
| Soybeans, canned, 1 cup | 1,180* |
| Canned sardines, 3½ ounces (100 g) | 1,190 |
| Canned pink salmon, 3½ ounces (100 g) | 980 |
| Canned tuna, 3½ ounces (100 g) | 560 |
| Egg, omega-3, 1 large | 145 |
| Egg, 1 large | 55 |

* Omega-3 fats in these foods are from ALA.

# IODINE SUPER FOODS

| FOOD | IODINE CONTENT*<br>(MICROGRAMS, MCG) |
| --- | --- |
| Cod, baked, 3 ounces (85 g) | 99 |
| Yogurt, plain, low-fat, 1 cup | 75 |
| Milk, low-fat, 1 cup | 56 |
| Bread, enriched, 2 slices | 45 |
| Fruit cocktail in heavy syrup, canned, ½ cup | 42 |
| Shrimp, 3 ounces (85 g) | 35 |
| Ice cream, chocolate, ½ cup | 30 |
| Egg, 1 large | 24 |
| Tuna, canned in oil, 3 ounces (85 g) | 17 |
| Cheese, cheddar, 1 slice | 12 |

* Approximate only (values depend on where the food is grown and how it is made)

Source: ods.od.nih.gov/factsheets/Iodine-HealthProfessional/

# VITAMIN D SUPER FOODS

| FOOD | VITAMIN D CONTENT<br>(MICROGRAMS, MCG) |
| --- | --- |
| Sardines, 3½ ounces (100 g) | 8.0 |
| Milk with added vitamin D, 1 cup | 5.0 |
| Soy milk with added vitamin D, 1 cup | 5.0 |
| Canned salmon, 3½ ounces (100 g) | 2.0 |
| Canned tuna, 3½ ounces (100 g) | 1.0 |
| Cheese, 1½ slices | 1.0 |
| Egg, 1 large | 0.5 |
| Milk, low-fat, 1 cup | 0.5 |
| Margarine, 2 teaspoons | 0.5 |
| Butter, 2 teaspoons | 0.1 |

# THE LOW GI EATING PLAN FOR AN OPTIMAL PREGNANCY: SUMMER MENU IDEAS

|  | BREAKFAST | MORNING SNACK | LUNCH |
|---|---|---|---|
| **MONDAY** | • Homemade Muesli (page 221) with plain yogurt and berries | • Peach<br>• Handful of almonds | • Vegetable Frittata (page 238)<br>• 1 slice of whole grain bread |
| **TUESDAY** | • Almond Butter & Banana (page 228) on 2 slices of whole grain toast | • Handful of dried apricots and almonds | • Salmon & Salad Whole Grain Sandwich (page 241)<br>• Kiwi |
| **WEDNESDAY** | • Berry Smoothie with Chia Seeds (page 226) | • Banana<br>• Handful of walnuts | • Avocado & Roasted Vegetable Whole Grain Wrap* (page 242) |
| **THURSDAY** | • Avocado and Tomato (page 228) on 2 slices of whole grain toast | • Mini Corn, Carrot & Zucchini Muffin (page 288) | • Chicken & Avocado Sandwich (page 241) on 2 slices of sourdough rye bread<br>• Nectarine |
| **FRIDAY** | • Homemade Muesli (page 221) with plain yogurt and kiwi | • Handful of dried apricots and almonds | • Falafel & Salad Whole Grain Wrap (page 242) |
| **SATURDAY** | • Tomato, Cheese & Spinach (page 229) on 2 slices of sourdough rye toast | • Berry Smoothie with Chia Seeds (page 226) | • Tuna Pasta Salad (page 235) |
| **SUNDAY** | • Apple & Buttermilk Pancakes with Blueberries & Yogurt (page 222) | • Sesame, Oat & Cranberry Cookie (page 287)<br>• Kiwi | • Homemade Burger (page 266)<br>• Orange |

**NOTE:** These meal plans are a guide only. While they have been designed to meet the nutritional needs of most women during pregnancy, as noted earlier in the book, it can be difficult to obtain the recommended intakes of iron, folate and iodine from dietary sources only, so supplements of these nutrients are generally recommended once you are trying to conceive. The amount of food you need to eat each day will also depend on whether you are pregnant, breastfeeding or trying to conceive and whether you are aiming to lose, maintain or gain weight, or manage your weight gain during pregnancy. For individualized advice, we recommend seeking the help of a registered dietitian.

| AFTERNOON SNACK | DINNER | EVENING SNACK |
|---|---|---|
| • Apple, Cinnamon & Ginger Muffin (page 280) | • Baked Chicken Breast with Ratatouille (page 256) | • Fruit & Nut Ball (page 284)<br>• Glass of low-fat milk or soy milk |
| • 2 Ryvitas® with Cottage Cheese & Sun-Dried Tomato (page 291) | • Tofu & Vegetable Pad Thai (page 244) | • Low-fat plain yogurt with berries, flaked almonds, sunflower seeds and pumpkin seeds |
| • Sesame, Oat & Cranberry Cookie (page 287) | • Ginger & Beef Soba Noodles (page 261) | • Glass of chocolate-flavored milk or soy milk<br>• 1 slice cinnamon raisin bread |
| • Plain low-fat yogurt with flaked almonds, pumpkin seeds and sunflower seeds | • Poached Salmon with Asian Greens (page 268) | • Mango, Kiwi & Lime Fruit Salad (page 286) |
| • 2 Ryvitas® with Avocado & Tomato (page 291) | • Chicken & Barley Risotto (page 255) | • Banana, Walnut & Fig Loaf (page 282)<br>• Glass of chocolate-flavored low-fat milk or soy milk |
| • Warm Chickpea & Carrot Dip (page 290) with vegetable crudités and toasted whole wheat pita bread | • Marinated Lamb Tenderloin with Mashed Sweet Potatoes (page 272) | • Fruit, Yogurt & Muesli Parfait (page 285) |
| • Fruit & Nut Ball (page 284)<br>• Glass of low-fat milk or soy milk | • Mexican Bean Tortillas with Avocado Salsa (paper 248) | • Peach Panna Cotta (page 277) |

# THE LOW GI EATING PLAN FOR AN OPTIMAL PREGNANCY: WINTER MENU IDEAS

|  | BREAKFAST | MORNING SNACK | LUNCH |
|---|---|---|---|
| MONDAY | • Banana & Coconut Oatmeal (page 220) | • Pear and handful of almonds | • Carrot, Ginger & Cannellini Bean Soup (page 232)<br>• 1 whole grain roll |
| TUESDAY | • Beans (page 229) on sourdough toast | • Berry Smoothie with Chia Seeds (page 226) | • Curried Egg Sandwich (page 241) on whole grain bread<br>• 1 kiwi |
| WEDNESDAY | • Homemade Muesli (page 221) with plain yogurt and berries | • Sesame, Oat & Cranberry Cookie (page 287) | • Tuna & Bean (page 242) whole grain wrap |
| THURSDAY | • Sardines (page 228) on 2 slices of whole grain toast<br>• Orange | • 2 Ryvitas® with Cottage Cheese & Sun-Dried Tomato (page 291) | • Chicken & Udon Noodle Soup with Asian Greens (page 233) |
| FRIDAY | • Banana & Coconut Oatmeal (page 220) | • Apple and handful of almonds | • Vegetarian Pita Pizza (page 239) |
| SATURDAY | • Scrambled Eggs (page 223) with whole grain English muffin<br>• Orange | • Sesame, Oat & Cranberry Cookie (page 287) | • Chicken Fillet Burger (page 240) |
| SUNDAY | • French Toast (page 227) | • Pear | • Vegetable Fried Rice (page 236) |

NOTE: These meal plans are a guide only. While they have been designed to meet the nutritional needs of most women during pregnancy, as noted earlier in the book, it can be difficult to obtain the recommended intakes of iron, folate and iodine from dietary sources only, so supplements of these nutrients are generally recommended once you are trying to conceive. The amount of food you need to eat each day will also depend on whether you are pregnant, breastfeeding or trying to conceive and whether you are aiming to lose, maintain or gain weight, or manage your weight gain during pregnancy. For individualized advice, we recommend seeking the help of a registered dietitian.

| AFTERNOON SNACK | DINNER | EVENING SNACK |
|---|---|---|
| • Banana, Walnut & Fig Loaf (page 282) | • Lentil & Vegetable Curry (page 246) with brown basmati rice | • Mug of warm chocolate-flavored milk or soy milk<br>• 1 slice cinnamon raisin bread |
| • 2 Ryvitas® with Peanut Butter & Banana (page 291) | • Meat Loaf with Roasted Vegetables (page 264) | • Cinnamon Baked Apples (page 275) with low-fat Greek yogurt |
| • Apple<br>• Glass of low-fat milk or soy milk | • Chicken Schnitzel with Baby Potatoes, Mushrooms & Arugula Salad (page 258) | • Handful of dried figs and almonds |
| • Fruit & Nut Ball (page 284)<br>• Glass of low-fat milk or soy milk | • Roasted Vegetable & Bean Lasagna (page 250) | • Mini Bread & Banana Pudding (page 276) |
| • Mini Corn, Carrot & Zucchini Muffin (page 288) | • Pork with Ginger Apples (page 260) | • Mug of warm chocolate-flavored milk or soy milk<br>• 1 slice of cinnamon raisin bread |
| • 2 Ryvitas® with almond butter<br>• Glass of low-fat milk or soy milk | • Baked Fish Packets with Sweet Potato Chips & Salad (page 270) | • Apple & Pear Crumble (page 274) with low-fat yogurt |
| • Low-fat plain yogurt with sliced banana, flaked almonds, sunflower seeds and pumpkin seeds | • Moroccan Chickpea & Vegetable Tagine (page 254) | • Banana, Walnut, & Fig Loaf (page 282) |

# PART 5
# Recipes

## LOW GI RECIPES FOR YOUR PREGNANCY JOURNEY

### BREAKFAST

### LIGHT MEALS

# MAIN DISHES

# DESSERTS

# SNACKS

## A NOTE ABOUT OVEN TEMPERATURES

All recipes in this book have been tested in convection ovens. The difference in temperature between conventional and convection (fan-forced) ovens is approximately 25 degrees Fahrenheit.

## OVEN TEMPERATURE CONVERSIONS

| FAHRENHEIT (CONVECTION) | FAHRENHEIT (CONVENTIONAL) | CELSIUS (CONVECTION) | CELSIUS (CONVENTIONAL) |
|---|---|---|---|
| 225° | 250° | 100° | 120° |
| 325° | 350° | 160° | 180° |
| 350° | 375° | 170° | 190° |
| 375° | 400° | 180° | 200° |
| 400° | 425° | 200° | 220° |
| 425° | 465° | 220° | 240° |
| 475° | 500° | 250° | 270° |

# Breakfast

# Banana & Coconut Oatmeal

Serves 2
Preparation time: 2 minutes
Cooking time: 5 minutes

⅔ cup (60 g) thick-cut rolled oats (not quick-cooking oats)
1 cup (250 ml) low-fat milk or soy milk
½ medium banana, sliced
1 heaping tablespoon raisins
1 teaspoon shredded coconut

1. Place the oats in a saucepan or large microwave-safe bowl. Add sufficient water to cover, plus about two thirds of the milk.
2. Bring to a boil and gently simmer for 3 minutes (or microwave) until thickened.
3. Add the sliced banana and cook for a further 1 to 2 minutes.
4. Add the remaining milk to make a smooth consistency and stir in the raisins.
5. Sprinkle with the coconut to serve.

**NUTRITIONAL ANALYSIS PER SERVING**
238 calories; Total fat 6 g; Saturated fat 3 g; Protein 9 g; Carbohydrates 35 g; Fiber 4 g; Sodium 56 mg; Iron 1.4 mg; Calcium 162 mg; Folate 49 mcg; ALA 57 mg; Long-chain omega-3 0 mg

# Homemade Muesli

This basic recipe is for a raw muesli, but if you prefer your muesli crunchy, see the toasted version below—ingredients are the same but oven-roasted.

Serves 8
Preparation time: 10 minutes
Cooking time: 25–30 minutes (for toasted variety)

2 cups (180 g) rolled oats
½ cup (70 g) sunflower seeds
¼ cup (70 g) pumpkin seeds
¼ cup (40 g) flaxseeds
¼ cup (30 g) sesame seeds
½ cup (30 g) shredded coconut
½ cup (80 g) raw peanuts
¼ cup (35 g) walnuts
½ cup (80 g) packed raisins
¼ cup (30 g) dried apricots, chopped

**For raw muesli**
1. Place all ingredients into a large mixing bowl. Stir to combine.
2. Store in an airtight container, and lightly shake the container before serving.
3. Serve with low-fat milk, soy milk or yogurt.

**For toasted muesli**
1. Preheat oven to 325°F/160°C.
2. Place the oats in a large baking dish and bake for 5 minutes.
3. Add the sunflower, pumpkin and flaxseeds and bake for a further 10 minutes.
4. Add the sesame seeds, coconut and nuts and bake for a further 10 to 15 minutes until the muesli is nicely brown and toasted. (Take care not to overcook.)
5. Allow the muesli to cool completely before adding the raisins and apricots.
6. Store in an airtight container and shake lightly before serving.
7. Serve with low-fat milk, soy milk or yogurt.

---

**NUTRITIONAL ANALYSIS PER SERVING**
384 calories; Total fat 25 g; Saturated fat 5 g; Protein 12 g; Carbohydrates 25 g; Fiber 8 g; Sodium 11 mg; Iron 3.8 mg; Calcium 58 mg; Folate 53 mcg; ALA 1,470 mg; Long-chain omega-3 0 mg

# Apple & Buttermilk Pancakes with Blueberries & Yogurt

Serves 2 (2 pancakes per serving)
Preparation time: 15 minutes
Cooking time: 20 minutes

¾ cup (120 g) whole wheat flour
¼ cup (40 g) all-purpose flour
1 tablespoon baking powder
5 ounces (140 g) unsweetened applesauce (about ½ cup plus
    1½ tablespoons)
1¼ cups (310 ml) buttermilk
2 large eggs
1 teaspoon vanilla extract
2 teaspoons reduced-fat tub margarine, melted
⅔ cup (180 g) low-fat vanilla yogurt
¾ cup (150 g) fresh blueberries

1. Sift the flours and baking powder into a large bowl. In a small bowl, whisk together the apple purée, buttermilk, eggs and vanilla extract until well combined.
2. Add the apple mixture to the flour mixture and mix until just combined.
3. Brush a nonstick skillet with the melted margarine. Heat over medium heat. Fry quarter-cupfuls of the batter in the skillet for 2 minutes on each side, or until cooked through. Wrap the cooked pancakes in a clean kitchen towel to keep them warm as you fry the remaining pancakes.
4. To serve, top with the yogurt and blueberries.

**NUTRITIONAL ANALYSIS PER SERVING**
301 calories; Total fat 6 g; Saturated fat 2 g; Protein 13 g; Carbohydrates 45 g; Fiber 5 g; Sodium 1,065 mg; Iron 1.3 mg; Calcium 280 mg; Folate 45 mcg; ALA 80 mg; Long-chain omega-3 19 mg

# Scrambled Eggs

Serves 1
Preparation time: 5 minutes
Cooking time: 5 minutes

1 teaspoon olive oil
2 large eggs
2 tablespoons plus 2 teaspoons low-fat or skim milk
Fresh chives, chopped
Freshly ground black pepper
1 whole grain English muffin, toasted, to serve

1. Heat the olive oil in a nonstick skillet.
2. Beat the eggs and milk until just mixed, and add to the pan on medium heat.
3. With a spatula, move the egg mixture around the pan until there is no raw egg visible.
4. Tip the eggs out onto a warm plate, scatter with the chives and black pepper and serve with the toasted whole grain muffin.

**COOK'S TIPS**

» The eggs start to set immediately and cook quickly, so you need to have the muffin already toasting.
» Some people like their scrambled eggs runny, but when you're pregnant, ensure that your eggs are cooked through.
» Scrambled eggs are good as part of a "big breakfast," especially with sautéed button mushrooms and grilled tomato halves (just skip the bacon and sausages!).

**NUTRITIONAL ANALYSIS PER SERVING**
379 calories; Total fat 19 g; Saturated fat 5 g; Protein 19 g; Carbohydrates 31 g; Fiber 3 g; Sodium 450 mg; Iron 3.8 mg; Calcium 203 mg; Folate 88 mcg; ALA 293 mg; Long-chain omega-3 84 mg

# Mushroom & Cheese Omelet

Serves 1
Preparation time: 5 minutes
Cooking time: 10 minutes

2 teaspoons olive oil
1 cup (100 g) sliced button mushrooms
1 tablespoon finely chopped chives (optional)
2 large eggs
1 tablespoon plus 1 teaspoon water
1 heaping tablespoon grated low-fat cheese
Extra chives, to serve
Freshly ground black pepper
1 slice whole wheat sourdough toast, to serve

1. Heat 1 teaspoon of the olive oil in a small nonstick skillet.
2. When hot, add the mushrooms in one layer, turning the heat down to low.
3. After 1 minute, add the chopped chives and cook a further 2 minutes, stirring.
4. Remove the mushrooms and wipe out the pan.
5. Heat the remaining oil in the pan.
6. Beat the eggs and water together.
7. Turn the heat to low and add the egg mixture, tilting the pan to distribute it around the pan.
8. After about 5 minutes, when the omelet starts to set, spread the mushrooms on one half of the omelet and sprinkle them with the grated cheese.
9. Once the omelet is completely set, with no raw or runny mixture visible, use a plastic spatula or a wooden spoon (or a combination) to loosen, and fold the omelet in half over the mushrooms.
10. Tip the omelet out onto a warm plate, scatter the omelet with chives and black pepper and serve with toast.

**NUTRITIONAL ANALYSIS PER SERVING**
406 calories; Total fat 23 g; Saturated fat 7 g; Protein 25 g; Carbohydrates 22 g; Fiber 5 g; Sodium 418 mg; Iron 3.4 mg; Calcium 212 mg; Folate 166 mcg; ALA 173 mg; Long-chain omega-3 91 mg

# Berry Smoothie with Chia Seeds

Serves 1
Preparation time: 3 minutes

1 tablespoon plus 1 teaspoon rolled oats
1 teaspoon chia seeds
1 cup strawberries or raspberries, fresh or frozen
½ cup low-fat milk
½ cup low-fat plain yogurt
2 teaspoons honey
A squeeze of lemon juice

Mix all the ingredients in a blender or using an immersion blender, and drink immediately. (If you wait, the mixture will get thicker and thicker, as the chia seeds contain highly viscous fiber.) Add more or less milk to your taste.

**NUTRITIONAL ANALYSIS PER SERVING**
310 calories; Total fat 5 g; Saturated fat 2 g; Protein 20 g; Carbohydrates 43 g; Fiber 8 g; Sodium 156 mg; Iron 3.2 mg; Calcium 448 mg; Folate 326 mcg; ALA 765 mg; Long-chain omega-3 724 mg

# French Toast

Serves 2
Preparation time: 2 minutes
Cooking time: 5 minutes

2 tablespoons canola oil
4 slices low GI whole grain bread
2 large eggs
2 tablespoons plus 2 teaspoons low-fat milk
2 tablespoons plus 2 teaspoons maple syrup, warmed
1 cup blueberries or strawberries, or one chopped banana, to serve

1. Heat 1 tablespoon of the oil on low heat in a nonstick skillet.
2. In a shallow bowl, lightly whisk the eggs and milk together.
3. Dip both sides of 2 slices of bread in the egg mixture.
4. Add both slices to the skillet and fry for 2 minutes, then flip and fry 2 minutes on the other side.
5. Transfer to a warmed plate. Heat the remaining tablespoon of oil in the pan and repeat steps 3 and 4 for the remaining 2 slices of bread.
6. To serve, trickle the warmed maple syrup over the toast and serve with the fruit.

> **NUTRITIONAL ANALYSIS PER SERVING (WITH BERRIES):**
> 400 calories; Total fat 16 g; Saturated fat 3 g; Protein 14 g; Carbohydrates 49 g; Fiber 4 g; Sodium 394 mg; Iron 2.4 mg; Calcium 132 mg; Folate 83 mcg; ALA 1024 mg; Long-chain omega-3 42 mg

# Toast Toppers

### ALMOND BUTTER & BANANA
Spread 2 slices of low GI whole grain toast with 1 tablespoon of almond butter, and top with a small sliced banana.

**NUTRITIONAL ANALYSIS PER SERVING**
281 calories; Total fat 10 g; Saturated fat 1 g; Protein 9 g, Carbohydrates 35 g; Fiber 5 g; Sodium 317 mg; Iron 1.8 mg; Calcium 106 mg; Folate 36 mcg; ALA 118 mg; Long-chain omega-3 0 mg

### AVOCADO & TOMATO
Spread 2 slices of low GI whole grain toast with half a small avocado, and top with 1 sliced tomato.

**NUTRITIONAL ANALYSIS PER SERVING**
290 calories; Total fat 13 g; Saturated fat 3 g; Protein 8 g, Carbohydrates 32 g; Fiber 7 g; Sodium 331 mg; Iron 1.9 mg; Calcium 89 mg; Folate 79 mcg; ALA 106 mg; Long-chain omega-3 0 mg

### SARDINES
Top 2 slices of low GI whole grain toast with a small can of sardines, and drizzle with fresh lemon juice.

**NUTRITIONAL ANALYSIS PER SERVING**
268 calories; Total fat 10 g; Saturated fat 3 g; Protein 16 g; Carbohydrates 28 g; Fiber 3 g; Sodium 608 mg; Iron 2.1 mg; Calcium 251 mg; Folate 20 mcg; ALA 310 mg; Long-chain omega-3 1215 mg

## BEANS

Combine ½ cup drained canned cannellini beans, 2 heaping tablespoons canned diced tomatoes and a sprinkle of finely chopped herbs (e.g., basil, thyme or chives). Warm in a saucepan or microwave and serve on 2 slices of sourdough toast.

### NUTRITIONAL ANALYSIS PER SERVING

317 calories; Total fat 3 g; Saturated fat 1 g; Protein 18 g; Carbohydrates 51 g; Fiber 14 g; Sodium 744 mg; Iron 5.2 mg; Calcium 189 mg; Folate 258 mcg; ALA 257 mg; Long-chain omega-3 0 mg

## MUSHROOMS

Sauté ¾ cup sliced button mushrooms for 1 to 2 minutes in 1 teaspoon of olive oil. Serve on 2 slices of whole wheat sourdough toast.

### NUTRITIONAL ANALYSIS PER SERVING

274 calories; Total fat 7 g; Saturated fat 1 g; Protein 9 g; Carbohydrates 40 g; Fiber 5 g; Sodium 373 mg; Iron 1.6 mg; Calcium 45 mg; Folate 189 mcg; ALA 120 mg; Long-chain omega-3 0 mg

## TOMATO, CHEESE & SPINACH

Spread 2 slices of rye sourdough toast with ½ cup of cottage cheese; top with 3 finely chopped sun-dried tomatoes and a large handful of baby spinach.

### NUTRITIONAL ANALYSIS PER SERVING

289 calories; Total fat 4 g; Saturated fat 1 g; Protein 14 g; Carbohydrates 45 g; Fiber 7 g; Sodium 453 mg; Iron 2.8 mg; Calcium 90 mg; Folate 198 mcg; ALA 108 mg; Long-chain omega-3 1 mg

# Light meals

# Carrot, Ginger & Cannellini Bean Soup

Provided by Kate Hemphill

Serves 10
Preparation time: 10 minutes
Cooking time: 20 minutes


3⅓ pounds (1.5 kg) carrots, scrubbed or peeled, ends trimmed and
    cut into 2-inch (5 cm) pieces
4-inch (10 cm) piece ginger, peeled and roughly chopped
2 large garlic cloves, peeled and roughly chopped
Chicken or vegetable stock to cover, about 3 cups (600 ml)
Two 14-ounce (400 g each) cans cannellini beans, rinsed and drained
    (3 cups)
1¼ cups (300 ml) light crème fraîche, or low-fat yogurt
Freshly ground black pepper


1. Put the carrots, ginger and garlic into a large saucepan; cover with the
   stock and bring to a boil, reduce the heat and gently simmer until the
   carrots are tender. Let cool 5 minutes.
2. Purée with an immersion blender or, carefully, in a blender, leaving some
   texture; then stir in the beans and crème fraîche. Add extra stock for a
   thinner soup.
3. Reheat, season with black pepper to taste and serve.

## COOK'S TIP
» If freezing, allow the soup to cool and ladle into 1- or 2-cup
  containers or ziplock bags for easy use.


**NUTRITIONAL ANALYSIS PER SERVING**
113 calories; Total fat 1 g; Saturated fat <1 g; Protein 7 g; Carbohydrates 16 g;
Fiber 9 g; Sodium 461 mg; Iron 1.3 mg; Calcium 147 mg; Folate 71 mcg;
ALA 58 mg; Long-chain omega-3 1 mg.

# Chicken & Udon Noodle Soup with Asian Greens

Serves 4
Preparation time: 15 minutes
Cooking time: 10 minutes

2 teaspoons olive oil
1½-inch (4 cm) piece fresh ginger, finely grated
2 garlic cloves, finely chopped
2 medium carrots, cut into short thin sticks
2 celery stalks, halved lengthwise, thinly sliced diagonally
2½ cups (625 ml) water
1½ cups (375 ml) reduced-sodium chicken stock
1 tablespoon plus 1 teaspoon reduced-sodium soy sauce
14 ounces (400 g) udon noodles
1 bunch bok choy, trimmed, cut into 1-inch (3 cm) pieces
2 cups finely shredded Chinese cabbage
12 ounces (350 g) skinless chicken breasts, trimmed of fat, thinly sliced
1 teaspoon sesame oil
Fresh cilantro leaves, to serve

1.  Heat the oil in a large saucepan over medium heat. Cook the ginger and garlic for 1 minute. Add the carrots and celery and cook, stirring often, for 2 minutes.
2.  Add the water, stock and soy sauce to the pan. Cover and bring to a simmer over medium heat. Add the noodles, bok choy and cabbage. Return to a simmer and cook, partially covered, for 2 minutes.
3.  Add the chicken and sesame oil to the pan. Cook for 1 to 2 minutes, until the chicken is cooked completely through.
4.  Divide the soup between serving bowls. Top with the cilantro to serve.

---

**NUTRITIONAL ANALYSIS PER SERVING**
318 calories; Total fat 6.5 g; Saturated fat 2 g; Protein 30 g; Carbohydrates 31 g; Fiber 7 g; Sodium 795 mg; Iron 3.1 mg; Calcium 160 mg; Folate 64 mcg; ALA 50 mg; Long-chain omega-3 13 mg.

# Barley & Chickpea Salad

Serves 4
Preparation time: 10 minutes (plus 6 hours soaking time)
Cooking time: 25 minutes (plus 30 to 60 minutes chilling time)

1 cup (200 g) pearl barley
3 cups (700 ml) water
One 14-ounce (400 g) can chickpeas, rinsed and drained
6 cups (60 g) baby spinach leaves
2 small English cucumbers, halved lengthwise, thinly sliced diagonally
1½ cups (250 g) cherry tomatoes, quartered or halved (9 ounces)
2 heaping tablespoons chopped dill
2 heaping tablespoons chopped flat-leaf parsley

**Yogurt dressing**
⅓ cup (60 g) low-fat Greek yogurt
1 teaspoon finely grated lemon zest
¼ lemon, juiced
1 teaspoon unhulled tahini (sesame paste)
2 teaspoons honey
¼ teaspoon ground smoked paprika
¼ teaspoon ground cumin
Freshly ground black pepper, to taste

1. In a large bowl, cover the barley with water and soak for 6 hours or overnight.
2. Drain the barley and add to a saucepan with the water. Bring to a boil, lower the heat and simmer for 20 minutes, or until tender. Drain the barley and rinse under cold water. Drain well and transfer to a large bowl.
3. Add the chickpeas, spinach, cucumbers, cherry tomatoes, dill and parsley. Toss to combine.
4. Whisk all the dressing ingredients together in a small bowl to make the dressing.
5. Add the yogurt dressing to the salad and toss to coat. If time allows, chill for 30 to 60 minutes to allow the flavors to meld before serving.

---

**NUTRITIONAL ANALYSIS PER SERVING**
294 calories; Total fat 5 g; Saturated fat 1 g; Protein 10 g; Carbohydrates 47 g; Fiber 11 g; Sodium 189 mg; Iron 3.9 mg; Calcium 115 mg; Folate 87 mcg; ALA 76 mg; Long-chain omega-3 2 mg

# Tuna Pasta Salad

Serves 2

Preparation time: 10 minutes (plus time to cook pasta and cool)

1 heaping tablespoon (20 g) pesto
3½ ounces (100 g) low-fat plain yogurt (about ½ small container)
One 5-ounce can tuna in springwater, drained (142 g)
1 cup cooled pasta (cooked according to package directions)
2 finely chopped shallots
½ medium red bell pepper (70 g), finely sliced
6 cherry tomatoes, halved
Freshly ground black pepper
2 cups mixed salad greens, to serve

1. Mix the pesto into the yogurt until well combined.
2. Mix the tuna, pasta, shallots, bell peppers and tomatoes in a large bowl, add the yogurt mixture and toss to combine.
3. Season with black pepper and serve on the salad greens.

---

**NUTRITIONAL ANALYSIS PER SERVING**
267 calories; Total fat 6 g; Saturated fat 1 g; Protein 22 g; Carbohydrates 29 g; Fiber 5 g; Sodium 242 mg; Iron 4.0 mg; Calcium 196 mg; Folate 115 mcg; ALA 4 mg; Long-chain omega-3 280 mg

# Vegetable Fried Rice

Serves 4
Preparation time: 20 minutes
Cooking time: 15 minutes

2 teaspoons canola or olive oil
2 large eggs, lightly beaten
1 large carrot, finely sliced
1 small head broccoli, cut into small florets
1 thumb-size piece ginger, grated
6 shallots, finely chopped
1 medium red bell pepper, chopped
1 cup (100 g) button mushrooms, sliced
1 medium zucchini, finely sliced
Half a 15-ounce (425 g) can whole baby corn
6 canned water chestnuts
1¼ cups (250 g) cooked brown rice, cooled
¼ teaspoon sesame oil
1 teaspoon reduced-sodium tamari or soy sauce
¼ cup (60 g) unsalted cashews, coarsely chopped, to serve

1. Heat a wok or skillet over high heat and add 1 teaspoon of the oil. When it is smoking slightly, add the eggs and swirl to create a thin omelet. When the omelet has set, turn to briefly cook the other side. Turn out and let cool, then roll up and cut into thin strips.
2. Blanch the carrot and broccoli in boiling water for 1 minute (or microwave briefly).
3. Add the remaining teaspoon of oil to the wok or skillet and heat to a moderately high temperature. Add the ginger, shallots and bell pepper and cook for 2 minutes, stirring constantly. Add the remaining vegetables, including the blanched carrot and broccoli, and stir-fry for a further 2 minutes, or until the vegetables are just softened.

4. Add the rice and egg strips and stir until well combined and heated through.
5. Season with the sesame oil and tamari and scatter the chopped cashews on top to serve.

### COOK'S TIP

» To save time, we used microwaveable brown rice, which cooks in 90 seconds.

### NUTRITIONAL ANALYSIS PER SERVING
295 calories; Total fat 13 g; Saturated fat 3 g; Protein 14 g; Carbohydrates 27 g; Fiber 8 g; Sodium 212 mg; Iron 2.9 mg; Calcium 64 mg; Folate 112 mcg; ALA 40 mg; Long-chain omega-3 21 mg

# Vegetable Frittata

Serves 4
Preparation time: 35 minutes (including 20 minutes cooling time)
Cooking time: 40 minutes

Olive oil cooking spray
One 14-ounce (400 g) butternut squash, peeled, seeded, and cut into
small cubes (11 ounces/310 g peeled weight)
2 teaspoons extra virgin olive oil
1½ cups (150 g) thickly sliced button mushrooms
2 cups (150 g) chopped broccoli
2 ears corn, kernels cut off (or 1 cup canned or frozen)
6 large eggs
¾ cup (185 ml) low-fat milk
Freshly ground black pepper
½ cup (60 g) 25% reduced-fat grated cheese, such as Cheddar

1. Preheat the oven to 375°F/180°C. Line an 8-cup (2-liter) ovenproof dish
   with parchment paper overhanging the sides.
2. Put the squash in a shallow microwave-safe dish with ¼ cup (60 ml)
   water. Cover and cook on high for 3 to 4 minutes, until the squash is
   tender. Drain and set aside.
3. Heat the olive oil in a large nonstick skillet over medium-high heat.
   Add the mushrooms, broccoli and corn. Cook, stirring often, for 3 to 4
   minutes, until the mushrooms start to soften. Remove the pan from the
   heat and set aside to cool for 10 minutes.
4. In a medium bowl, whisk the eggs, milk and black pepper together.
5. Put all the vegetables in a large bowl and toss gently to combine. Transfer
   to the lined dish and pour the egg mixture on top.
6. Sprinkle on the cheese. Bake for 30 to 35 minutes, until set and golden
   brown. Let cool in the baking dish for 10 minutes before cutting into
   pieces and serving.

---

**NUTRITIONAL ANALYSIS PER SERVING**
326 calories; Total fat 16 g; Saturated fat 6 g; Protein 24 g; Carbohydrates 19 g;
Fiber 8 g; Sodium 217 mg; Iron 2.7 mg; Calcium 235 mg; Folate 145 mcg;
ALA 94 mg; Long-chain omega-3 70 mg

# Vegetarian Pita Pizzas

Serves 4
Preparation time: 5 minutes
Cooking time: 3 minutes

8 small whole wheat pitas
2 tablespoons plus 2 teaspoons prepared (store-bought) pizza sauce or
    tomato purée
2 cups cherry tomatoes, halved
1 red or yellow bell pepper, sliced
One 8-ounce can (225 g) kidney beans (1 scant cup)
½ cup sliced olives
½ cup grated mozzarella cheese
Dried thyme and oregano, for sprinkling

1. Preheat the broiler to high (475°F/250°C).
2. Spread the pizza sauce onto the pitas and top with the cherry tomatoes, bell pepper, kidney beans and olives.
3. Sprinkle with the cheese and herbs.
4. Cook the pizzas under the broiler until the cheese melts and the pizzas are warmed through (the base should be crisp), about 3 minutes.

**NUTRITIONAL ANALYSIS PER SERVING**
507 calories; Total fat 11 g; Saturated fat 4 g; Protein 20 g; Carbohydrates 74 g;
Fiber 15 g; Sodium 1,177 mg; Iron 5.9 mg; Calcium 220 mg; Folate 92 mcg;
ALA 247 mg; Long-chain omega-3 8 mg

# Chicken Fillet Burger

Serves 4
Preparation time: 10 minutes (plus 30 minutes marinating time)
Cooking time: 8 minutes

1 tablespoon plus 1 teaspoon olive oil
1 tablespoon plus 1 teaspoon lemon juice
1 heaping tablespoon freshly ground black pepper
1 heaping tablespoon chopped herbs (flat-leaf parsley, thyme or chives)
Two 9-ounce (250 g each) chicken breasts, halved horizontally (so they are thinner)
Olive oil cooking spray
4 whole grain rolls, to serve
1 medium avocado, halved and pitted
1 large English cucumber, trimmed and cut into thin slices, lengthwise
2 cups (25 g) baby spinach (loosely packed)
2 tomatoes, sliced

1. Combine the oil, lemon juice, pepper and herbs. Add the chicken and stir to coat. Cover and refrigerate for 30 minutes to marinate.
2. Heat a lightly oiled grill pan or skillet. Cook the chicken over high heat for 2 minutes on each side, or until completely cooked through.
3. Split the bread rolls in half. Spread each half with avocado.
4. Divide the cucumber, spinach and tomato between the rolls. Add the chicken fillets and top with remaining roll halves.

**Alternative option**
1. Cook the chicken breasts whole for 5 minutes on each side, or until cooked through, and slice.
2. To serve, pile the chicken on top of salad greens tossed with a small amount of balsamic or red wine vinegar. Serve with whole grain bread or wraps.

---

**NUTRITIONAL ANALYSIS PER SERVING**
478 calories; Total fat 22 g; Saturated fat 5 g; Protein 36 g; Carbohydrates 31 g; Fiber 7 g; Sodium 378 mg; Iron 3.2 mg; Calcium 133 mg; Folate 89 mcg; ALA 160 mg; Long-chain omega-3 18 mg

# Sandwiches

## CURRIED EGG

Mash 1 hard-boiled egg with 1 heaping tablespoon of plain Greek yogurt and ½ teaspoon of curry powder. Place on 2 slices of low GI multigrain bread with chopped lettuce.

**NUTRITIONAL ANALYSIS PER SERVING**

267 calories; Total fat 8 g; Saturated fat 3 g; Protein 13 g; Carbohydrates 32 g; Fiber 5 g; Sodium 373 mg; Iron 3.4 mg; Calcium 140 mg; Folate 133 mcg; ALA 133 mg; Long-chain omega-3 42 mg

## SALMON & SALAD

Fill 2 slices of low GI multigrain bread with one 3¾ -ounce (106 g) can of salmon (drained), half of a sliced English cucumber and ½ cup of baby spinach.

**NUTRITIONAL ANALYSIS PER SERVING**

320 calories; Total fat 10 g; Saturated fat 3 g; Protein 25 g; Carbohydrates 29 g; Fiber 4 g; Sodium 823 mg; Iron 2.9 mg; Calcium 415 mg; Folate 128 mcg; ALA 200 mg; Long-chain omega-3 2,260 mg

## CHICKEN & AVOCADO

Spread 2 slices of rye sourdough bread with a quarter of an avocado and fill with 1½ ounces (50 g) poached chicken breast (sliced), half a sliced English cucumber and a handful of baby spinach.

**NUTRITIONAL ANALYSIS PER SERVING**

348 calories; Total fat 9 g; Saturated fat 2 g; Protein 23 g; Carbohydrates 40 g; Fiber 5 g; Sodium 398 mg; Iron 2.0 mg; Calcium 67 mg; Folate 203 mcg; ALA 100 mg; Long-chain omega-3 9 mg

# Wraps

### FALAFEL & SALAD
Spread 1 multigrain low GI wrap with 1 heaping tablespoon of hummus and top with 2 crushed or sliced falafel, half of a sliced English cucumber and ½ cup of shredded lettuce. Roll up to serve.

**NUTRITIONAL ANALYSIS PER SERVING**
219 calories; Total fat 8 g; Saturated fat 1 g; Protein 7 g; Carbohydrates 23 g; Fiber 12 g; Sodium 315 mg; Iron 2.6 mg; Calcium 59 mg; Folate 38 mcg; ALA 48 mg; Long-chain omega-3 0 mg

### TUNA & BEAN
Combine one 3½-ounce (95 g) can of tuna (drained) with 1 heaping tablespoon plain Greek yogurt, ¼ cup of cannellini beans (rinsed and drained), half of a diced English cucumber and 2 slices of finely chopped Spanish onion. Spread on 1 multigrain low GI wrap, and roll up to serve.

**NUTRITIONAL ANALYSIS PER SERVING**
284 calories; Total fat 5 g; Saturated fat 2 g; Protein 30 g; Carbohydrates 25 g; Fiber 10 g; Sodium 544 mg; Iron 2.9 mg; Calcium 92 mg; Folate 55 mcg; ALA 98 mg; Long-chain omega-3 535 mg

### AVOCADO & ROASTED VEGETABLES
Cut a quarter of a red bell pepper, 1 small zucchini, 1 small baby eggplant and a quarter of a medium sweet potato into thin slices; arrange on a baking sheet and brush or spray with olive oil. Bake at 375°F/180°C until cooked to your liking (test with a knife after 15 minutes). (These can be made the previous night and stored in the fridge.) Spread a wrap with half a small avocado and top with the roasted vegetables before wrapping.

**NUTRITIONAL ANALYSIS PER SERVING**
313 calories; Total fat 17 g; Saturated fat 4 g; Protein 7 g; Carbohydrates 28 g; Fiber 12 g; Sodium 88 mg; Iron 2.2 mg; Calcium 65 mg; Folate 90 mcg; ALA 59 mg; Long-chain omega-3 0 mg

# Main dishes

# Tofu & Vegetable Pad Thai

Serves 4
Preparation time: 15 minutes
Cooking time: 15 minutes

One 6-ounce package (150 g) dried rice noodles
2 teaspoons olive oil
2 large eggs, lightly beaten
One 7-ounce (200 g) baby eggplant, halved lengthwise and thinly sliced
2 cups (200 g) cauliflower, cut into small florets
1 yellow bell pepper, cut into short thin strips
2 cups (125 g) snow peas (4½ ounces), cut into thin strips
1¼ cups (125 g) thinly sliced button mushrooms
1 medium red onion, cut into thin wedges
2 garlic cloves, finely chopped
1 tablespoon plus 1 teaspoon sweet chili sauce
2 tablespoons plus 2 teaspoons freshly squeezed lime juice
1 heaping tablespoon brown sugar
1 teaspoon fish sauce
7 ounces (200 g) marinated tofu, cut into strips
½ cup cilantro
2 tablespoons chopped unsalted peanuts

1. Soak the noodles in boiling water for 5 minutes. Drain well and set aside.
2. Heat 1 teaspoon of the oil in a large wok over medium-high heat. Add the eggs and swirl to coat the wok. Cook for 2 to 3 minutes, until the eggs are set. Transfer to a plate.
3. Heat the remaining oil in the wok over medium-high heat. Stir-fry the eggplant, cauliflower, bell pepper, snow peas, mushrooms, onion and garlic for 2 to 3 minutes, until the vegetables are tender but still crisp.
4. Meanwhile, whisk the sweet chili sauce, lime juice, brown sugar and fish sauce together in a small bowl.
5. Add the noodles, tofu and sauce mixture to the vegetables. Toss to combine and heat through. Top with the cilantro and chopped peanuts.

## NUTRITIONAL ANALYSIS PER SERVING

277 calories; Total fat 13 g; Saturated fat 2 g; Protein 16 g; Carbohydrates 19 g; Fiber 10 g; Sodium 276 mg; Iron 3.5 mg; Calcium 222 mg; Folate 116 mcg; ALA 250 mg; Long-chain omega-3 22 mg

# Lentil & Vegetable Curry

Serves 4
Preparation time: 10 minutes
Cooking time: 20 minutes

1¼ cups (270 g) dried red lentils
1 tablespoon olive oil
1 medium yellow onion, finely chopped
2 celery stalks, chopped
2 garlic cloves, finely chopped
1-inch (3 cm) piece fresh ginger, finely grated
2 teaspoons ground cilantro
1 teaspoon ground turmeric
1 teaspoon ground cumin
One 13.5-ounce (400 ml) can light coconut milk
1½ cups (375 ml) reduced-sodium chicken or vegetable stock
2 medium zucchini, chopped
1½ cups (150 g) broccoli, cut into small florets
1½ cups (150 g) cauliflower, cut into small florets
1 large carrot, chopped
3 cups (100 g) baby spinach

1.  Put the lentils in a fine colander and rinse under cold water. Heat the oil in a large saucepan over medium heat. Add the onion, celery, garlic and ginger. Cook, stirring often, for 3 minutes, or until the vegetables soften.
2.  Add the cilantro, turmeric and cumin and cook for 1 minute. Add the lentils and cook for a further 2 minutes. Stir in the coconut milk and stock. Cover and bring to a simmer. Reduce heat to medium-low and cook, partially covered, for 5 minutes.
3.  Add the zucchini, broccoli, cauliflower and carrot. Cook, covered, for 10 minutes, or until the vegetables are tender. Remove the pan from the heat and stir in the spinach. Stir until the spinach wilts.

---

**NUTRITIONAL ANALYSIS PER SERVING**
380 calories; Total fat 15 g; Saturated fat 8 g; Protein 23 g; Carbohydrates 33 g;
Fiber 16 g; Sodium 434 mg; Iron 8.9 mg; Calcium 156 mg; Folate 185 mcg;
ALA 250 mg; Long-chain omega-3 5 mg

# Bowties 'n' Beans

Provided by Johanna Burani

Makes five 1-cup servings
Preparation time: 10 minutes
Cooking time: 10 minutes

1 tablespoon extra virgin olive oil
2 garlic cloves, minced
6 cups (175 g) fresh spinach, each leaf and stem quartered
6 oil-packed sun-dried tomatoes, coarsely chopped
One 14-ounce (400 g) can cannellini beans, drained and rinsed (1½ cups)
Pinch of dried thyme
Black pepper
½ cup hot water
2 cups uncooked farfalle (bowtie or butterfly) pasta
1 tablespoon oil from sun-dried tomatoes jar
2 heaping tablespoons grated pecorino romano cheese

1. Warm the olive oil in a large heavy saucepan. Add the garlic and spinach and sauté on medium-high heat for 4 to 5 minutes, until the spinach is wilted. Add the sun-dried tomatoes (reserving the oil), beans, thyme, black pepper and hot water. Reduce the heat and simmer for 5 minutes.
2. In the meantime, cook the pasta according to package directions until al dente.
3. Drain the pasta, and add it to the sauce in the pan. Drizzle the oil from the sun-dried tomatoes jar over the pasta and, using tongs, mix well. Serve immediately with the grated cheese on the side for sprinkling on top.

---

**NUTRITIONAL ANALYSIS PER SERVING**
307 calories; Total fat 10 g; Saturated fat 2 g; Protein 11 g; Carbohydrates 41 g; Fiber 7 g; Sodium 554 mg; Iron 3.5 mg; Calcium 94 mg; Folate 81 mcg; ALA 165 mg; Long-chain omega-3 2 mg

# Mexican Bean Tortillas with Avocado Salsa

Serves 8
Preparation time: 12 minutes
Cooking time: 15 minutes

### Bean mixture

1 tablespoon canola oil
1 red onion, finely chopped
2 garlic cloves, crushed
1 teaspoon chili paste
1 teaspoon coriander
One 14-ounce (400 g) can diced tomatoes
One 14-ounce (400 g) can cannellini beans, rinsed and drained
One 14-ounce (400 g) can refried beans

### Salsa

1 large avocado, chopped
1 small red onion, chopped
1 small tomato, chopped
½ cup fresh cilantro, chopped
1 English cucumber, chopped
1 tablespoon canola oil
½ lemon, juiced

### To serve

8 corn tortillas
½ cup low-fat plain yogurt (optional)

1. Heat the oil in a skillet over medium heat. Add the onion, garlic, chili paste and coriander, and cook for 3 to 4 minutes, until the onion is softened.
2. Add the tomatoes and beans. Simmer for 10 to 12 minutes, stirring occasionally.
3. Combine and toss all the salsa ingredients in a medium bowl.
4. Serve the bean mixture with salsa and tortillas.
5. Add a dollop of plain yogurt if desired.

**NUTRITIONAL ANALYSIS PER SERVING (WITH YOGURT)**
233 calories; Total fat 12 g; Saturated fat 2 g; Protein 8 g; Carbohydrates 19 g; Fiber 8 g; Sodium 409 mg; Iron 2.2 mg; Calcium 116 mg; Folate 62 mcg; ALA 513 mg; Long-chain omega-3 0 mg

# Roasted Vegetable & Bean Lasagna

Serves 4

Preparation time: 20 minutes

Cooking time: 1 hour (plus 10 minutes resting)

Olive oil cooking spray

1¼ pound (600 g) butternut squash, peeled, seeded, thinly sliced

1 large eggplant, thinly sliced lengthwise

2 large zucchini, thickly sliced lengthwise

2 tablespoons olive oil

2 cups (500 g) part-skim fresh ricotta

2 large eggs

½ cup (125 ml) low-fat milk

Freshly ground black pepper, to taste

One 14-ounce (400 g) jar tomato sauce, or 14-ounce (400 g) can no-salt-added tomato purée (low-sodium option)

10 to 12 fresh lasagna noodles (150 g) or no-boil lasagna noodles

One 14-ounce (400 g) can cannellini beans, rinsed and drained

5 cups (150 g) baby spinach

½ cup (60 g) coarsely grated 25% reduced-fat cheddar cheese

1. Preheat the oven to 425°F/220°C. Coat a 10-cup (2.5-liter) ovenproof dish with cooking spray. Line a large roasting pan with parchment paper. Toss the squash, eggplant, zucchini and oil together in a large bowl. Spread out over the roasting pan. Roast for 30 minutes, or until the vegetables are very tender. Reduce the oven temperature to 375°F/180°C.
2. Whisk the ricotta, eggs, milk and black pepper together in a large bowl.
3. Spread a little of the pasta sauce over the bottom of the ovenproof dish. Top with a layer of lasagna noodles, cutting to fit if necessary. Spoon one third of the sauce over the pasta. Top with one third of the roasted vegetables and one third of the beans followed by the spinach. Spread with about one third of the ricotta mixture.

4. Repeat the layering with another third of the pasta, sauce, vegetables, beans, spinach and half of the remaining ricotta. Top with a final layer of the pasta, sauce, vegetables, beans, spinach and pasta. Spoon the remaining ricotta over the top and sprinkle with the cheddar cheese.
5. Bake for 30 minutes, or until the pasta is tender when tested with a small knife. (If using dry, no-boil noodles, this may take longer.) Let cool for 10 minutes before cutting.

**NUTRITIONAL ANALYSIS PER SERVING**
487 calories; Total fat 18 g; Saturated fat 7 g; Protein 34 g; Carbohydrates 41 g; Fiber 12 g; Sodium 931 mg; Iron 4.2 mg; Calcium 639 mg; Folate 205 mcg; ALA 300 mg; Long-chain omega-3 33 mg

# Lentil & Vegetable Shepherd's Pie

Serves 4
Preparation time: 15 minutes
Cooking time: 1 hour

3 teaspoons olive oil
1 medium yellow onion, chopped
2 celery stalks, chopped
2 carrots, chopped
1¼ cups (125 g) button mushrooms, sliced
1 cup fresh or frozen corn kernels
1 cup (210 g) dried French-style (puy or green) lentils, rinsed
1 teaspoon dried rosemary leaves
2 cups (500 ml) water
One 14-ounce (400 g) can no-salt-added tomato purée
½ cup (125 ml) reduced-sodium vegetable stock
3 tablespoons chopped flat-leaf parsley
1 pound (500 g) sweet potatoes, peeled and chopped
1 pound (500 g) new potatoes, peeled and chopped
½ cup (60 g) 25% reduced-fat grated cheese, such as Cheddar

1. Heat the oil in a large saucepan over medium heat. Add the onion, celery, carrots, mushrooms and corn. Cook, uncovered, stirring often, for 6 to 7 minutes, or until softened slightly.
2. Add the lentils, rosemary, water, tomato purée and stock to the vegetables. Cover and bring to a simmer. Cook, covered, over low heat for 30 minutes, or until the lentils are tender. Remove from the heat and let cool for 10 minutes; then stir in the parsley and pour into an ovenproof dish.
3. Preheat the oven to 350°F/190°C.

4. Meanwhile, cook the sweet potatoes and new potatoes in a large saucepan of boiling water for 12 to 15 minutes, until very tender. Drain and mash.
5. Spoon the mashed potatoes over the lentil mixture and rough up the surface with a fork. Sprinkle with the cheese and bake for 20 minutes, or until the cheese melts.

**NUTRITIONAL ANALYSIS PER SERVING**
507 calories; Total fat 10 g; Saturated fat 3 g; Protein 28 g; Carbohydrates 69 g; Fiber 18 g; Sodium 335 mg; Iron 7.3 mg; Calcium 283 mg; Folate 156 mcg; ALA 164 mg; Long-chain omega-3 8 mg

# Moroccan Chickpea & Vegetable Tagine

Serves 4
Preparation time: 10 minutes
Cooking time: 15 minutes

2 teaspoons olive oil
1 medium yellow onion, cut into thin slivers
1 garlic clove, finely chopped
3 teaspoons Moroccan seasoning *(ras el hanout)*
One 1¼-pound (600 g) butternut squash, peeled, seeded and chopped
2 cups (200 g) cauliflower, cut into small florets
One 14-ounce (400 g) can no-salt-added tomatoes
½ cup (125 mL) reduced-sodium vegetable stock
2 cups (200 g) broccoli florets
One 14-ounce (400 g) can chickpeas, rinsed and drained
1 cup (200 g) quinoa, rinsed well
Cilantro, to serve
Lemon zest, to serve

1. Heat the oil in a large saucepan over medium heat. Add the onion and garlic and cook for 4 to 5 minutes, until the onion softens. Stir in the Moroccan seasoning and cook for 1 minute.
2. Stir in the squash, cauliflower, tomatoes and stock. Cook, covered, for 10 minutes. Add the broccoli and chickpeas and cook, covered, for a further 5 minutes, or until the vegetables are tender.
3. Meanwhile, put the rinsed quinoa in a saucepan and cover with 2 cups water. Bring to a boil, then reduce the heat and simmer for 10 minutes, or until the grains are tender and translucent.
4. Divide the quinoa between serving bowls. Top with the tagine, cilantro and lemon zest.

---

**NUTRITIONAL ANALYSIS PER SERVING**
165 calories; Total fat 8 g; Saturated fat 1 g; Protein 18 g; Carbohydrates 57 g; Fiber 14 g; Sodium 379 mg; Iron 7.8 mg; Calcium 144 mg; Folate 206 mcg; ALA 120 mg; Long-chain omega-3 2 mg

# Chicken & Barley Risotto

Serves 4
Preparation time: 15 minutes (plus 6 hours soaking time)
Cooking time: 40 minutes

1¼ cups (250 g) pearl barley
2 teaspoons olive oil
1 pound (400 g) skinless chicken thighs, trimmed of fat
1 leek, halved lengthwise, thinly sliced
2 medium carrots, finely chopped
1 garlic clove, crushed
1½ cups (375 ml) water
1¼ cups (310 ml) reduced-sodium chicken stock
One 14-ounce (400 g) can no-salt-added diced tomatoes
2 cups (125 g) snow peas (4½ ounces), diagonally sliced
1 cup (130 g) frozen peas
1 bunch asparagus, woody ends trimmed, diagonally sliced
½ cup (30 g) finely grated Parmesan

1. Soak the barley in cold water for 6 hours or overnight. Drain.
2. Heat 1 teaspoon of the oil in a large saucepan over medium-high heat. Add the chicken thighs and cook for 3 to 4 minutes on each side, until just cooked. Transfer to a plate. Set aside to cool, then thinly slice.
3. Heat the remaining oil in the pan over medium heat. Add the leek, carrots and garlic. Cook for 5 to 6 minutes, stirring often, until the leek starts to soften.
4. Add the water, stock, tomatoes and drained barley to the saucepan and stir. Cover and bring to a simmer. Take the lid off and cook, uncovered, for 20 to 25 minutes, until the barley is almost tender. Stir occasionally to prevent sticking.
5. Stir the snow peas, frozen peas, asparagus and cooked chicken into the pan. Cook for a further 5 to 10 minutes, until the vegetables are tender but still crisp. Serve sprinkled with the Parmesan.

---

**NUTRITIONAL ANALYSIS PER SERVING**
492 calories; Total fat 16 g; Saturated fat 5 g; Protein 31 g; Carbohydrates 49 g; Fiber 15 g; Sodium 642 mg; Iron 4.5 mg; Calcium 178 mg; Folate 111 mcg; ALA 160 mg; Long-chain omega-3 28 mg

# Baked Chicken Breast with Ratatouille

Recipe modified from *Australian Healthy Food Guide*, July 2009

Serves 4
Preparation time: 10 minutes
Cooking time: 20 minutes

1 large zucchini, cut into 1-inch (2 cm) cubes
1 large red bell pepper, seeded, cut into 1-inch (2 cm) cubes
1 large onion
1 small eggplant (300 g), cut into 1-inch (2 cm) cubes
1 tablespoon canola oil
Freshly ground black pepper
Four 5-ounce (150 g each) skinless chicken breasts
3½ ounces (100 g) sun-dried tomatoes, cut into strips
One 15-ounce (420 g) can cannellini beans, rinsed and drained
2 teaspoons dried mixed herbs
2 teaspoons fresh thyme leaves
Balsamic vinegar, to serve

1. Preheat the oven to 400°F/200°C.
2. Toss the zucchini, bell pepper, onion and eggplant in a large bowl with half the oil and some black pepper.
3. Spread out onto a large baking sheet and bake for 10 to 12 minutes.
4. Heat the remaining oil in a nonstick skillet. Cook the chicken for 2 to 3 minutes on each side, until golden brown.
5. Remove the vegetables from the oven. Add the sun-dried tomatoes and cannellini beans to the sheet and sprinkle with the dried herbs and fresh thyme.
6. Place the chicken breasts in a single layer on top of the vegetables and season with more black pepper.
7. Return the baking sheet to the oven and roast for a further 10 minutes, or until the chicken is cooked through.

8. To serve, divide the vegetables between four plates. Top each with a piece of chicken and drizzle with a little balsamic vinegar.

**COOK'S TIP**

» Be careful to cook chicken sufficiently; it should never be pink inside.

**NUTRITIONAL ANALYSIS PER SERVING**

324 calories; Total fat 5 g; Saturated fat 1 g; Protein 42 g; Carbohydrates 21 g; Fiber 11 g; Sodium 252 mg; Iron 4.0 mg; Calcium 120 mg; Folate 105 mcg; ALA 316 mg; Long-chain omega-3 20 mg

# Chicken Schnitzel with Baby Potatoes, Mushrooms & Arugula Salad

Serves 4
Preparation time: 10 minutes
Cooking time: 20 minutes

2 tablespoons plus 2 teaspoons flour
Two 9-ounce (250 g each) chicken breasts, halved horizontally
1 large egg, beaten
1 cup homemade dry bread crumbs (see Cook's Tip)
Olive oil cooking spray
8 new potatoes
2 cups (200 g) button mushrooms
1 teaspoon olive oil
2 cups arugula
¼ sliced red onion
1 red bell pepper, cut into thin strips
2 cups grape or cherry tomatoes, halved
2 teaspoons balsamic vinegar
½ cup (40 g) shaved Parmesan cheese

1. Preheat the oven to 375°F/180°C.
2. Place the flour in a large plastic bag, add the chicken breasts, and shake to coat. Shake off any surplus flour.
3. Dip the chicken in the beaten egg and then in the bread crumbs.
4. Lightly coat a baking sheet with olive oil cooking spray, and bake the chicken for 20 minutes, turning after 10. Take care not to overcook, but check that the chicken is not pink at all (see Cook's Tip).
5. While the chicken bakes, steam the potatoes in a steamer basket set in a pot filled with 1 inch of boiling water for 10 minutes, or until cooked.
6. Sauté the mushrooms in the olive oil on very low heat.
7. Place the arugula in a salad bowl with the onion, bell pepper and tomatoes. Sprinkle with the balsamic vinegar and toss. Top with the shaved Parmesan.
8. To serve, divide the chicken, potatoes and mushrooms between four plates. Serve with the salad.

## COOK'S TIPS

- » Chicken breasts often come with the tenderloins attached underneath. Separate these before slicing the chicken into the two fillets, and coat separately. They will only need half the cooking time.
- » To make bread crumbs, slowly dry whole grain bread slices in the oven for 20 minutes at 225°F/100°C; then pulse in a food processor when cool.
- » To ensure the chicken is cooked through, make a small cut halfway through the thickest part of the schnitzel; it should not be pink at all.

**NUTRITIONAL ANALYSIS PER SERVING**

282 calories; Total fat 9 g; Saturated fat 4 g; Protein 43 g; Carbohydrates 38 g; Fiber 6 g; Sodium 421 mg; Iron 3.0 mg; Calcium 193 mg; Folate 133 mcg; ALA 118 mg; Long-chain omega-3 34 mg

# Pork with Ginger Apples

Serves 4
Preparation time: 10 minutes
Cooking time: 20 minutes

3 medium apples, peeled and cored, thinly sliced
2-inch (4 cm) piece fresh ginger, peeled, finely grated
1 teaspoon finely grated lemon zest
⅓ cup (80 ml) water
1 teaspoon olive oil
Four ¼-pound (125 g each) pork loin chops, trimmed of all visible fat
Freshly ground black pepper
1¼ pounds (600 g) new potatoes, halved and steamed, to serve
4 medium zucchini, halved lengthwise, diagonally sliced and steamed, to serve
4 cups (250 g) snow peas (9 ounces), trimmed and steamed, to serve

1. Put the apple slices, ginger, lemon zest and water in a medium saucepan. Cook, covered, over medium heat for 12 to 15 minutes, until the apple slices are just tender.
2. While the apple slices are cooking, heat the oil in a large nonstick skillet over medium heat. Season the pork with the black pepper and add to the pan. Cook for 2 minutes on each side. Transfer to a plate, cover with foil, and set aside for a few minutes to rest.
3. Serve the pork with the ginger apples and vegetables.

**NUTRITIONAL ANALYSIS PER SERVING**
338 calories; Total fat 3 g; Saturated fat 1 g; Protein 35 g; Carbohydrates 37 g; Fiber 8 g; Sodium 67 mg; Iron 3 mg; Calcium 55 mg; Folate 157 mcg; ALA 20 mg; Long-chain omega-3 15 mg

# Ginger & Beef Soba Noodles

Serves 4
Preparation time: 15 minutes
Cooking time: 15 minutes

1 teaspoon cornstarch

2 tablespoons plus 2 teaspoons reduced-sodium soy sauce

2 tablespoons plus 2 teaspoons rice wine vinegar

1 tablespoon plus 1 teaspoon sweet chili sauce

1 tablespoon plus 1 teaspoon freshly squeezed lime juice

1 teaspoon olive oil

1 pound (500 g) lean top round steak, trimmed of fat and thinly sliced across the grain

One 14-ounce (400 g) package fresh or frozen stir-fry vegetables

2 cups (200 g) cremini mushrooms, thinly sliced

2 cups (200 g) broccoli, cut into small florets

2 garlic cloves, finely chopped

2-inch (4 cm) piece ginger, coarsely grated

One 12.7-ounce (360 g) package soba noodles, cooked according to package directions and drained

2 tablespoons cilantro

1.  Put the cornstarch into a small bowl and whisk in the soy sauce, vinegar, sweet chili sauce and lime juice until smooth.
2.  Heat ½ teaspoon of the oil in a wok on high heat until very hot. Add half the steak and stir-fry for 30 to 60 seconds, until browned. Use a slotted spoon to transfer the cooked meat to a plate. Repeat with the remaining steak.
3.  Add the remaining oil to the wok and reheat until hot. Add the stir-fry vegetables, mushrooms, broccoli, garlic and ginger. Stir-fry for 2 minutes, or until the vegetables are tender but still crisp.
4.  Add the sauce mixture and noodles to the wok, and toss until well combined and heated through. Return the meat to the wok and toss to combine and heat through.
5.  Divide the wok contents between bowls, and garnish with the cilantro to serve.

---

**NUTRITIONAL ANALYSIS PER SERVING**
388 calories; Total fat 9 g; Saturated fat 3 g; Protein 38 g; Carbohydrates 33 g; Fiber 11 g; Sodium 625 mg; Iron 5 mg; Calcium 70 mg; Folate 58 mcg; ALA 110 mg; Long-chain omega-3 89 mg

# Asian Noodles with Lemongrass Meatballs

Serves 4
Preparation time: 15 minutes
Cooking time: 15 minutes

1 pound (500 g) ground skinless chicken
2 garlic cloves, crushed
1 egg white (from 1 large egg), lightly whisked
2 tablespoons chopped cilantro
2-inch (4 cm) piece ginger, finely grated
2 teaspoons olive oil
2 tablespoons reduced-sodium soy sauce
2 tablespoons sweet chili sauce
1 stalk lemongrass, white part only, finely chopped
1 medium green bell pepper, thinly sliced
1 medium zucchini, halved lengthwise and thinly diagonally sliced
4 baby eggplants, thinly diagonally sliced
1 cup (100 g) shiitake mushrooms (stems removed), sliced
½ cup (115 g) baby corn, halved lengthwise
1 bunch bok choy, trimmed, cut into 2-inch (4 cm) lengths
14 ounces (400 g) udon noodles, cooked according to package
     directions and drained

1.  To make the meatballs, combine the ground chicken, garlic, egg white,
    cilantro and ginger in a bowl. Shape teaspoonfuls of the mixture into
    small balls. Heat 1 teaspoon of the oil in a large nonstick skillet over
    medium heat. Add the meatballs and cook for 2 to 3 minutes, turning
    occasionally, until just cooked. Transfer to a plate and set aside.
2.  In a small bowl, mix together the soy and chili sauces.

3. Heat the remaining teaspoon of oil in a large wok until hot. Add the lemongrass, bell pepper, zucchini, eggplant, mushrooms, corn and bok choy to the wok. Stir-fry for 3 minutes, or until the vegetables are tender but still crisp.
4. Add the noodles, sauce mixture and meatballs to the wok. Toss until combined and heated through.

**NUTRITIONAL ANALYSIS PER SERVING**
430 calories; Total fat 15 g; Saturated fat 4 g; Protein 37 g; Carbohydrates 33 g; Fiber 9 g; Sodium 756 mg; Iron 4.7 mg; Calcium 149 mg; Folate 93 mcg; ALA 159 mg; Long-chain omega-3 48 mg

# Meat Loaf with Roasted Vegetables

Serves 4
Preparation time: 20 minutes
Cooking time: 60 minutes

Cooking oil spray
1 pound (500 g) lean ground beef
1 slice whole grain bread, made into crumbs (about ¾ cup of fresh bread crumbs)
1 medium onion or 6 shallots, finely chopped
1 medium carrot, grated
1 medium zucchini, grated
1 medium apple, peeled and grated
1 large egg, lightly beaten
One 15-ounce (425 g) can lentils , rinsed and drained
1 tablespoon sweet chili sauce, for glazing
2 medium new potatoes, peeled and cut into quarters
One 7-ounce (200 g) butternut squash, peeled and cut into 2-inch (4 cm) cubes
4 small onions, peeled
1 tablespoon olive oil
1¾ cups (200 g) green beans
1 cup (130 g) frozen peas

1. Preheat the oven to 375°F/180°C, and spray a baking pan with cooking oil spray.
2. Put the ground beef, bread crumbs, onion, carrot, zucchini, apple, egg and lentils into a large bowl and mix well to combine.
3. In the bowl, shape the mixture into a ball, tip into the prepared baking pan and mold into a loaf shape.
4. Bake for 60 minutes, brushing with the sweet chili sauce after 40 minutes.
5. While the meat loaf is baking, toss the potato, squash and onion in the olive oil on a separate baking sheet and bake in the oven for 30 minutes, or until cooked.

6. Steam the green beans and peas in a steamer basket set in a pot filled with 1 inch of boiling water for 5 minutes, or until cooked.
7. Slice the meat loaf and serve with the roasted vegetables and steamed vegetables.

## NUTRITIONAL ANALYSIS PER SERVING

530 calories; Total fat 19 g; Saturated fat 6 g; Protein 42 g; Carbohydrates 40 g; Fiber 15 g; Sodium 249 mg; Iron 6.2 mg; Calcium 130 mg; Folate 103 mcg; ALA 170 mg; Long-chain omega-3 61 mg

# Homemade Burgers

Serves 6
Preparation time: 15 minutes
Cooking time: 20 minutes

2½ teaspoons olive oil
½ large onion, finely chopped
1 garlic clove, finely chopped
1 pound (500 g) lean ground beef
1 large egg
1 cup rolled oats
1 tablespoon reduced-sodium soy sauce
6 whole grain rolls
2 cups salad greens
6 slices canned beets
1 avocado, sliced
Freshly ground black pepper

1. Heat 1 teaspoon of the olive oil in a nonstick skillet. Gently sauté the onion and garlic until transparent, about 5 minutes.
2. In a large bowl, combine the ground beef, cooked onion and garlic, egg, rolled oats and soy sauce.
3. Using slightly moistened hands, shape the mixture into six patties.
4. Cook the burgers either on the grill, on a lightly greased grill pan or in a nonstick skillet in the remaining 1½ teaspoons oil until cooked through, about 10 minutes on each side.
5. Serve on rolls with the salad greens and sliced vegetables. Sprinkle with black pepper to taste.

**NUTRITIONAL ANALYSIS PER SERVING**
519 calories; Total fat 22 g; Saturated fat 6 g; Protein 31 g; Carbohydrates 47 g;
Fiber 8 g; Sodium 878 mg; Iron 6.9 mg; Calcium 160 mg; Folate 196 mcg;
ALA 210 mg; Long-chain omega-3 33 mg

# Salmon Patties

Serves 4
Preparation time: 15 minutes (plus 30 minutes resting time)
Cooking time: 10 minutes

1⅓ cups (250 g) cooked brown rice

Half a 14.75-ounce can (210 g) pink salmon, drained and skin removed

4 shallots, finely chopped

1 large egg, lightly beaten

2 slices of whole grain bread, made into bread crumbs (about 1½ cups of
   fresh crumbs)

1 heaping tablespoon chopped fresh flat-leaf parsley

Zest and juice of half a lemon, other half cut into wedges for garnish

1 tablespoon olive or canola oil

2 medium carrots, sliced

4 medium zucchini, sliced

3¾ cups (200 g) snow peas (7 ounces), trimmed

1. Combine the rice with the salmon, shallots, egg, bread crumbs and
   parsley in a large bowl.
2. Add the lemon zest and juice to the salmon mixture.
3. Refrigerate the mixture for 30 minutes before dividing it into 8 portions.
4. Using slightly moistened hands, shape the portions into patties.
5. Heat the oil in a nonstick skillet over medium heat, and cook the patties
   until golden, approximately 5 minutes on each side.
6. Meanwhile, steam the carrots, zucchini, and snow peas in a steamer
   basket set in a pot with 1 inch of boiling water for 5 minutes, or until
   cooked.
7. Serve the patties with the lemon wedges and steamed vegetables.

---

**NUTRITIONAL ANALYSIS PER SERVING**
296 calories; Total fat 10 g; Saturated fat 2 g; Protein 16 g; Carbohydrates 32 g;
Fiber 6 g; Sodium 277 mg; Iron 2.2 mg; Calcium 150 mg; Folate 55 mcg;
ALA 200 mg; Long-chain omega-3 743 mg

# Poached Salmon with Asian Greens with a Soy & Sesame Dressing

Serves 4
Preparation time: 15 minutes
Cooking time: 15 minutes

1½ cups (375 ml) water
1 cup (250 ml) reduced-sodium chicken stock
Few sprigs dill
Few slices lemon
4 black peppercorns
Four 5-ounce (150 g each) pieces skinless and boneless salmon fillets
1 cup (210 g) Uncle Ben's Converted rice
2 bunches Chinese broccoli (*gai lan*), ends trimmed
2 tablespoons plus 2 teaspoons freshly squeezed lime juice
1 tablespoon plus 1 teaspoon reduced-sodium soy sauce
1 teaspoon sesame oil
1 garlic clove, crushed
1 heaping tablespoon sesame seeds, toasted (see Cook's Tip)

1. Put the water, stock, dill, lemon and peppercorns in a medium nonstick skillet and bring to a gentle simmer. Add the salmon and cover with a round of parchment paper. Cook over low heat, turning the salmon over once, for 8 to 10 minutes, until the salmon is just cooked. Using a slotted spoon, transfer the salmon to a plate.
2. While the salmon is cooking, cook the rice in a saucepan of boiling water, following package directions, or until tender. Drain.
3. Steam the Chinese broccoli over medium heat in a steamer basket set in a pot filled with 1 inch of boiling water for 3 to 4 minutes, until tender.

4. Whisk the lime juice, soy sauce, sesame oil and garlic together in a small bowl.
5. To serve, divide the rice and Chinese broccoli between plates. Place the salmon on top of the rice, drizzle with the soy mixture and sprinkle with the sesame seeds.

### COOK'S TIP

» To toast the sesame seeds, add them to a small nonstick skillet, and cook over medium heat, stirring often, for 3 to 4 minutes, until lightly toasted.

**NUTRITIONAL ANALYSIS PER SERVING**
527 calories; Total fat 19 g; Saturated fat 5 g; Protein 42 g; Carbohydrates 43 g; Fiber 4 g; Sodium 511 mg; Iron 4.8 mg; Calcium 108 mg; Folate 14 mcg; ALA 130 mg; Long-chain omega-3 2,953 mg

# Baked Fish Packets with Sweet Potato Chips & Salad

Serves 4
Preparation time: 10 minutes
Cooking time: 15 minutes

4 cups (75 g) baby spinach, washed and drained
Four 6-ounce (180 g each) thick white fish fillets (e.g., cod or snapper)
1¾ ounces (50 g ) oil-packed sun-dried tomatoes, drained and cut into strips
Zest of 1 lemon
¼ teaspoon chili powder
¼ teaspoon freshly ground black pepper
2 tablespoons olive oil
Olive oil cooking spray
2 medium new potatoes, peeled and cut into thin slices
7 ounces (200 g) sweet potato, peeled and cut into thin slices
2 carrots, peeled and cut into diagonal slices
2 cups (200 g) broccoli florets
1 cup (100 g) green beans
4 lemon wedges, for serving

1.  Preheat the oven to 425°F/220°C.
2.  Cut four 15-inch (38 cm) square sheets of aluminum foil and divide the spinach between them. Season the fish with the sun-dried tomatoes, lemon zest, chili powder and black pepper, and place on top of the spinach. Sprinkle the oil onto the fish.
3.  Bring the two sides of the foil to meet in the middle and crimp the foil from the middle to the edges, shaping it into a half moon.
4.  Fold the foil over again and crimp again so that no air can escape. Repeat for the other three packets.
5.  Bake for 15 minutes on a baking sheet; the packets will puff up like balloons.

6. While the fish is cooking, spray a baking sheet and the potato, sweet potato and carrot slices with olive oil cooking spray. Arrange the vegetables on the baking sheet, and bake for 10 to 15 minutes, until cooked.
7. Steam the broccoli and beans in a steamer basket set in a pot filled with 1 inch of boiling water for 7 to 8 minutes, until cooked.
8. To serve, snip open the packets and slide the fish onto plates. Serve with the lemon wedges and the steamed vegetables.

**NUTRITIONAL ANALYSIS PER SERVING**
390 calories; Total fat 12 g; Saturated fat 2 g; Protein 41 g; Carbohydrates 26 g; Fiber 9 g; Sodium 215 mg; Iron 4.6 mg; Calcium 107 mg; Folate 121 mcg; ALA 109 mg; Long-chain omega-3 319 mg

# Marinated Lamb Tenderloin with Mashed Sweet Potatoes

Serves 4

Preparation time: 15 minutes (plus 2 hours or overnight for marinating)

Cooking time: 20 minutes

2 tablespoons plus 2 teaspoons balsamic vinegar

1 tablespoon plus 1 teaspoon extra virgin olive oil

1 heaping tablespoon finely chopped rosemary leaves

2 garlic cloves, crushed

Freshly ground black pepper

1 pound (500 g) lamb tenderloins, trimmed of fat and sinew

2¼ pounds (1 kg) sweet potato, peeled and chopped (about 800 g peeled)

8 cups (800 g) broccoli and cauliflower florets

1.  To make the marinade, combine the vinegar, oil, rosemary, garlic and black pepper in a shallow dish. Add the lamb and turn in the marinade to coat. Cover and refrigerate for 2 hours, or overnight, to marinate.
2.  Cook the sweet potato in a large saucepan of boiling water for 10 minutes, or until very tender. Drain well. Mash until smooth.
3.  Preheat a griddle over medium heat. Drain the marinade off the lamb. Cook the lamb for 1½ to 2 minutes on each side for medium doneness. Transfer to a plate and set aside for a few minutes to rest. (Alternatively, follow the same steps to grill the lamb outdoors.)
4.  Steam the broccoli and cauliflower florets.
5.  Slice the lamb across the grain. Put the sweet potato mash on plates. Top with the sliced lamb and any pan juices, and serve with the steamed vegetables.

---

**NUTRITIONAL ANALYSIS PER SERVING**

411 calories; Total fat 13 g; Saturated fat 3 g; Protein 38 g; Carbohydrates 31 g; Fiber 11 g; Sodium 149 mg; Iron 5.7 mg; Calcium 112 mg; Folate 95 mcg; ALA 120 mg; Long-chain omega-3 93 mg

# Desserts

# Apple & Pear Crumble

Serves 4
Preparation time: 5 minutes
Cooking time: 40 minutes

2 apples, peeled and sliced
2 pears, peeled and sliced
1 tablespoon olive-oil-based butter substitute
2 heaping tablespoons all-purpose flour
2 heaping tablespoons brown sugar
1 teaspoon cinnamon (optional)
1 heaping tablespoon sunflower seeds
⅓ cup rolled oats
⅓ cup desiccated coconut
Low-fat ice cream, for serving (optional)

1. Preheat the oven to 375°F/180°C.
2. Place the apple and pear slices into a saucepan with 1 cup of water and cook for about 20 minutes.
3. Spoon the apple and pear mixture into one large or four individual ovenproof dishes.
4. In a small bowl, combine the olive oil spread, flour, brown sugar and cinnamon (if using), and rub with your fingertips until incorporated and crumbly.
5. Add the seeds, oats and coconut and mix well.
6. Top the apple and pear mixture with the crumble, pressing down firmly.
7. Bake for 15 to 20 minutes, until golden.
8. Serve with low-fat ice cream if desired.

**NUTRITIONAL ANALYSIS PER SERVING (WITHOUT ICE CREAM)**
285 calories; Total fat 11 g; Saturated fat 5 g; Protein 3 g; Carbohydrates 39 g;
Fiber 8 g; Sodium 25 mg; Iron 1.4 mg; Calcium 37 mg; Folate 48 mcg;
ALA 240 mg; Long-chain omega-3 3 mg

# Cinnamon Baked Apples

Serves 2
Preparation time: 5 minutes
Cooking time: 40 minutes

2 red or green apples
2 heaping tablespoons walnuts, finely chopped
2 heaping tablespoons sliced almonds
2 heaping tablespoons raisins
½ teaspoon cinnamon
2 teaspoons brown sugar
Greek yogurt, to serve

1. Preheat the oven to 375°F/180°C.
2. Wash and core the apples. Place them upright in a lightly oiled baking dish.
3. In a bowl, combine the walnuts, almonds, raisins, cinnamon and brown sugar. Mix well.
4. Stuff each apple with the nut mixture.
5. Cover the dish with foil and bake for 35 to 45 minutes, until the apples are tender when poked with a toothpick.
6. Remove the dish from the oven, and place an apple on each plate. Spoon the cooking liquid from the baking dish over the apples and serve immediately with a dollop of Greek yogurt on each.

**NUTRITIONAL ANALYSIS PER SERVING (WITHOUT YOGURT)**
281 calories; Total fat 12 g; Saturated fat 1 g; Protein 5 g; Carbohydrates 36 g; Fiber 6 g; Sodium 9 mg; Iron 1.4 mg; Calcium 61 mg; Folate 95 mcg; ALA 544 mg; Long-chain omega-3 0 mg

# Mini Bread & Banana Puddings

Recipe provided by Lisa Taylor, Gestational Diabetes Recipes
gestationaldiabetesrecipes.com

Serves 4
Preparation time: 10 minutes
Cooking time: 35 to 40 minutes

1 tablespoon light cooking oil

2 cups skim milk

2 large eggs

2 small bananas, mashed

1 teaspoon vanilla extract

1 teaspoon ground cinnamon

6 slices low GI seed or multigrain bread, crusts removed, halved
    diagonally

½ cup blueberries (frozen or fresh)

Reduced-fat ice cream, for serving (optional)

1. Preheat the oven to 350°F/170°C.
2. Lightly grease one baking dish or four individual ramekins with oil. Set aside.
3. Whisk together the milk, eggs, mashed banana, vanilla extract and cinnamon in a large bowl until combined.
4. Soak each piece of bread in the milk mixture for a few seconds.
5. Place four of the bread triangles in the baking dish or one in each individual ramekin, scatter with one third of the blueberries, then spread with the milk mixture. Repeat the layering process until all the bread triangles have been used.
6. Pour any remaining milk mixture and blueberries over the top, then sprinkle lightly with a little more cinnamon.
7. Bake for 35 to 40 minutes, until puffed and golden. Serve with a small dollop of ice cream if desired.

---

**NUTRITIONAL ANALYSIS PER SERVING (WITHOUT ICE CREAM)**
260 calories; Total fat 6 g; Saturated fat 1 g; Protein 13 g; Carbohydrates 37 g;
Fiber 6 g; Sodium 320 mg; Iron 3 mg; Calcium 220 mg; Folate 57 mcg;
ALA 12 mg; Long-chain omega-3 18 mg

# Peach Panna Cotta

Serves 4
Preparation time: 10 minutes
Refrigeration time: 3 hours or overnight

7 ounces (200 ml) low-fat evaporated milk (about half a can)
¼ cup sugar
1½ teaspoons powdered gelatin
6 ounces (200 ml) low-fat peach yogurt (1 container)
Fresh peach slices, for serving

1. Heat the milk and sugar in a saucepan over low heat until the sugar has dissolved.
2. Pour ½ cup of the mixture into a small cup or bowl and the remainder into a medium mixing bowl.
3. Sprinkle the gelatin into the ½ cup of milk, add to a double boiler and whisk over simmering water until incorporated.
4. Mix the yogurt into the milk in the bowl, then add the gelatin mixture.
5. Pour into greased coffee cups or small ramekins, and refrigerate for several hours, or overnight, until firm.
6. Dip the ramekins quickly into very hot water to loosen the panna cotta for serving, or loosen with a knife before turning out onto plates. Serve with fresh peach slices to garnish.

### COOK'S TIP
» As serving sizes are quite small, double the quantities to serve six for a larger dessert.

### NUTRITIONAL ANALYSIS PER SERVING
148 calories; Total fat 1 g; Saturated fat .5 g; Protein 8 g; Carbohydrates 28 g; Fiber 0 g; Sodium 87 mg; Iron 0.2 mg; Calcium 217 mg; Folate 4 mcg; ALA 1 mg; Long-chain omega-3 1 mg

# Snacks

# Apple, Cinnamon & Ginger Muffins

Makes 12
Preparation time: 10 minutes
Cooking time: 20 minutes

Cooking oil spray
1 cup (160 g) whole wheat flour
½ cup (75 g) all-purpose flour
½ cup (45 g) rolled oats
1 tablespoon baking powder
2 heaping tablespoons oat bran
2 tablespoons plus 2 teaspoons packed dark brown sugar
1 teaspoon ground cinnamon
1 teaspoon ground ginger
2 large eggs
5 ounces (140 g) unsweetened applesauce (about ⅔ cup)
⅔ cup (170 ml) low-fat milk
2 tablespoons (40 g) low- or no-trans-fat canola oil spread, melted
2 medium apples, peeled and coarsely grated

1. Preheat the oven to 350°F/ 170°F. Line a 12-cup muffin pan with paper baking cups and coat lightly with cooking oil spray.
2. In a large bowl, combine the flours, oats, baking powder, bran, brown sugar, cinnamon and ginger.
3. In a medium bowl, whisk together the eggs, apple purée, milk and melted spread.

4. Add the egg mixture and grated apple to the flour mixture, and mix until just combined. Divide the mixture evenly among the muffin cups, and bake for 18 to 20 minutes, until a toothpick inserted into one of the muffins comes out clean. Remove from the oven and transfer to a wire rack. Serve warm or at room temperature.

**COOK'S TIP**

» These muffins will keep in an airtight container at room temperature for up to two days.
» To freeze, wrap the muffins individually in plastic wrap, and then freeze in sealed freezer bags or an airtight container for up to two months. Thaw at room temperature.

**NUTRITIONAL ANALYSIS PER SERVING (1 MUFFIN)**
46 calories; Total fat 3 g; Saturated fat 1 g; Protein 4 g; Carbohydrates 24 g; Fiber 3 g; Sodium 160 mg; Iron 1.1 mg; Calcium 48 mg; Folate 33 mcg; ALA 11 mg; Long-chain omega-3 7 mg

# Banana, Walnut & Fig Loaf

Serves 12

Preparation time: 15 minutes (plus 20 minutes standing time)
Cooking time: 45 minutes (plus 10 minutes standing time)

Cooking oil spray
¾ cup (100 g) dried figs, finely chopped
2 tablespoons firmly packed dark brown sugar
1 teaspoon baking soda
½ cup (125 ml) boiling water
½ cup (130 g) low-fat vanilla yogurt
2 large eggs
2 tablespoons extra light olive oil, or canola oil
2 medium ripe bananas, mashed
1 cup (150 g) all-purpose flour
2 teaspoons baking powder
2 tablespoons plus 2 teaspoons wheat germ
⅓ cup (45 g) walnuts, finely chopped
Light cream cheese (Neufchâtel), to spread (optional)

1. Preheat the oven to 350°F/ 170°C. Line the bottom and two long sides of an 8½ x 4-inch loaf pan with parchment paper.
2. Put the dried figs and brown sugar in a medium heatproof bowl. Sprinkle with the baking soda and pour in the boiling water. Stir and set aside for 20 minutes.
3. In a small bowl, whisk together the yogurt, eggs and oil, then stir in the mashed bananas.
4. In another small bowl, combine the flour, baking powder and wheat germ.

5.  Stir the walnuts and the yogurt mixture into the fig mixture. Add the flour mixture and stir until well combined. Pour the batter into the loaf pan and smooth the surface. Bake for 40 to 50 minutes, until a toothpick inserted into the center of the loaf comes out clean. Remove from the oven and let cool in the pan for 10 minutes, then turn out onto a wire rack to cool completely.
6.  Slice the loaf and serve warm or at room temperature, spread with a little cream cheese, if you like.

**COOK'S TIP**

»   To freeze, wrap slices of the loaf individually in plastic wrap, and then freeze in sealed freezer bags or an airtight container for up to two months. Thaw at room temperature.

**NUTRITIONAL ANALYSIS PER SERVING (1 SLICE WITHOUT CREAM CHEESE)**

168 calories; Total fat 7 g; Saturated fat 1 g; Protein 5 g; Carbohydrates 21 g; Fiber 3 g; Sodium 224 mg; Iron 0.7 mg; Calcium 57 mg; Folate 22 mcg; ALA 28 mg; Long-chain omega-3 7 mg

# Fruit & Nut Balls

Makes 18 balls (2 balls per serving)
Preparation time: 15 minutes

½ cup (60 g) finely chopped dried apricots
½ cup (40 g) roughly chopped dried apples
½ cup (60 g) pitted prunes
3 tablespoons FSA mix (see Cook's Tip)
2 teaspoons unhulled tahini (sesame paste)

1. Pulse the apricots, apples, prunes and FSA mix in a food processor until the fruit is finely chopped. Add the tahini and process until well combined. The mixture will be very thick.
2. Shape teaspoonfuls of the mixture into balls, making 18 in total. Place in a container lined with wax paper and keep in the fridge.

### COOK'S TIP

» Keep these fruit and nut balls in an airtight container in the fridge for up to two weeks.
» To make your own FSA mix, combine 3 cups of flaxseeds, 2 cups of sunflower seeds, and 1 cup of almonds in a food processor and pulse to a fine meal. Store in the fridge in an airtight container.

### NUTRITIONAL ANALYSIS PER SERVING (2 BALLS)

73 calories; Total fat 3 g; Saturated fat 0 g; Protein 2 g; Carbohydrates 9 g; Fiber 3 g; Sodium 9 mg; Iron 0.6 mg; Calcium 22 mg; Folate 4 mcg; ALA 320 mg; Long-chain omega-3 0 mg

# Fruit, Yogurt & Muesli Parfait

Serves 4

Preparation time: 5 minutes

21 ounces (600 g) low-fat plain yogurt (about 2½ cups)

1 large mango, sliced

1¼ cups (200 g) strawberries, sliced

½ cup (50 g) toasted muesli (see recipe on page 221)

1. Take four glasses and spoon about ¼ cup (75 g) of yogurt into the bottom of each one. Divide the mango slices between the glasses; then top with a thin layer of toasted muesli.
2. Add another layer of yogurt, then the strawberries and, finally, the rest of the toasted muesli. Serve immediately, so the muesli stays crunchy.

**COOK'S TIP**

» If mango and strawberries are unavailable, replace them with frozen berries, sliced banana or sliced kiwi.

**NUTRITIONAL ANALYSIS PER SERVING**

179 calories; Total fat 4 g; Saturated fat 1 g; Protein 13 g; Carbohydrates 19 g; Fiber 3 g; Sodium 134 mg; Iron 1.2 mg; Calcium 371 mg; Folate 84 mcg; ALA 245 mg; Long-chain omega-3 0 mg

# Mango, Kiwi & Lime Fruit Salad

Adapted from Kate Hemphill

Serves 2
Preparation time: 5 minutes

½ cup (100 ml) mango purée
Pinch of ground ginger
1 lime, juiced
2 ripe kiwi
2 ripe mangoes, peeled and diced

1. Combine the mango purée, ginger and lime juice in a small bowl.
2. Cut each kiwi in half and spoon the pulp into a bowl. Add the diced mango and stir in the mango-lime dressing.

**NUTRITIONAL ANALYSIS PER SERVING**
158 calories; Total fat .5 g; Saturated fat 0 g; Protein 3 g; Carbohydrates 35 g; Fiber 7 g; Sodium 7 mg; Iron 1 mg; Calcium 38 mg; Folate 134 mcg; ALA 10 mg; Long-chain omega-3 0 mg

# Sesame, Oat & Cranberry Cookies

Makes 12
Preparation time: 10 minutes (plus 10 minutes standing time)
Cooking time: 20 minutes

2 cups (180 g) rolled oats
⅓ cup (50 g) dried cranberries, finely chopped
¼ cup (40 g) whole wheat flour
½ teaspoon baking powder
2 heaping tablespoons sunflower seeds
¼ cup honey
2 heaping tablespoons unhulled tahini (sesame paste)
1 large egg

1. Preheat the oven to 350°F/170°C. Line two baking sheets with parchment paper.
2. In a medium bowl, combine the oats, cranberries, flour, baking powder and sunflower seeds.
3. In a small bowl, whisk the honey, tahini and egg.
4. Add the honey mixture to the oat mixture and mix until well combined.
5. Spoon small tablespoonfuls of the mixture onto the lined baking sheets about 1 inch (3 cm) apart. Use the back of a spoon to press out slightly.
6. Bake for 20 minutes or until golden brown. Remove from the oven and let cool on the sheets for 10 minutes before transferring to a wire rack to cool completely.

## COOK'S TIP
» These cookies will keep in an airtight container at room temperature for up to four days.

## NUTRITIONAL ANALYSIS PER SERVING (1 COOKIE)
146 calories; Total fat 5 g; Saturated fat 1 g; Protein 4 g; Carbohydrates 20 g; Fiber 3 g; Sodium 33 mg; Iron 1.0 mg; Calcium 27 mg; Folate 12 mcg; ALA 3 mg; Long-chain omega-3 4 mg

# Mini Corn, Carrot & Zucchini Muffins

Makes 36 (3 per serving)
Preparation time: 10 minutes
Cooking time: 15 minutes

Cooking oil spray
1 cup (160 g) whole wheat flour
2 teaspoons baking powder
2 tablespoons plus 2 teaspoons wheat germ
⅓ cup (35 g) finely grated Parmesan
½ teaspoon olive oil
½ cup (70 g) fresh or frozen corn kernels
1 medium carrot, finely grated
1 large zucchini, coarsely grated, moisture squeezed out
1 cup (300 g) silken tofu, mashed until smooth
¼ cup (60 ml) low-fat milk
2 large eggs

1.  Preheat the oven to 350°F/ 170°C. Line three 1¾ x ¾-inch (30 ml) mini muffin pans with paper baking cups. Coat the cups with cooking oil spray.
2.  In a medium bowl, combine the flour, baking powder, wheat germ and Parmesan.
3.  Heat the oil in a medium nonstick skillet over medium-high heat. Cook the corn, carrot and zucchini for 4 to 5 minutes, stirring often, until the vegetables soften. Set aside to cool slightly.
4.  In a large bowl, mash the tofu with a fork until almost smooth (you could blend in a small food processor or with an immersion blender if you prefer). Add the milk and eggs. Whisk well to combine.
5.  Add the flour mixture and vegetables to the tofu mixture and mix until just combined. Spoon the mixture evenly into the muffin cups.
6.  Bake the muffins for 15 minutes, or until a toothpick inserted into a muffin comes out clean. Remove from the oven and let cool in the pan for 5 minutes before transferring to a wire rack to cool completely.

**COOK'S TIP**

» Keep the muffins in an airtight container in the fridge for up to four days. You can warm them slightly in the oven or microwave before serving, if you like.

» To freeze, wrap a serving of three muffins in plastic wrap and freeze in sealed freezer bags or an airtight container for up to two months. Thaw at room temperature.

**NUTRITIONAL ANALYSIS PER SERVING (3 MUFFINS)**
104 calories; Total fat 3 g; Saturated fat 1 g; Protein 6 g; Carbohydrates 12 g; Fiber 3 g; Sodium 153 mg; Iron 1.1 mg; Calcium 61 mg; Folate 26 mcg; ALA 6 mg; Long-chain omega-3 9 mg

# Warm Chickpea & Carrot Dip

Serves 4
Preparation time: 5 minutes
Cooking time: 15 minutes

2 cups (400 g) carrots, cut into 1-inch (2 cm) pieces
One 14-ounce (400 g) can chickpeas, rinsed and drained
⅓ cup (90 g) 2% plain yogurt
2 teaspoons curry powder or curry paste
Pinch of chili powder
2 tablespoons chopped fresh cilantro
Raw vegetables cut into sticks, to serve (e.g., carrots and celery)

1. Cook the carrots in a large saucepan of boiling water over medium heat for 5 minutes, or until tender, then drain and return to the pan.
2. Add the chickpeas, yogurt and curry powder, and mash until just combined.
3. Season with the chili powder, cover and keep warm.
4. Spoon the dip into a serving bowl and sprinkle with cilantro to garnish.
5. Serve with the raw vegetable sticks.

**NUTRITIONAL ANALYSIS PER SERVING (DIP ONLY)**
64 calories; Total fat 1 g; Saturated fat 0 g; Protein 3 g; Carbohydrates 9 g; Fiber 4 g; Sodium 115 mg; Iron 1.0 mg; Calcium 63 mg; Folate 31 mcg; ALA 24 mg; Long-chain omega-3 0 mg

# Ryvita® Crispbreads with Toppings

## COTTAGE CHEESE & SUN-DRIED TOMATO

Top 2 Ryvitas® (Pumpkin Seeds & Oats or Sunflower Seeds & Oats) with ½ cup of cottage cheese mixed with 2 finely chopped sun-dried tomatoes and chopped chives.

**NUTRITIONAL ANALYSIS PER SERVING**

140 calories; Total fat 3 g; Saturated fat 1 g; Protein 8 g; Carbohydrates 18 g; Fiber 5 g; Sodium 177 mg; Iron 1.6 mg; Calcium 50 mg; Folate 9 mcg; ALA 40 mg; Long-chain omega-3 1 mg

## AVOCADO & TOMATO

Top 2 Ryvitas® (Pumpkin Seeds & Oats or Sunflower Seeds & Oats) with half of a small avocado and 1 medium sliced tomato.

**NUTRITIONAL ANALYSIS PER SERVING**

149 calories; Total fat 6 g; Saturated fat 1 g; Protein 4 g; Carbohydrates 16 g; Fiber 6 g; Sodium 110 mg; Iron 1.3 mg; Calcium 26 mg; Folate 49 mcg; ALA 22 mg; Long-chain omega-3 0 mg

## PEANUT BUTTER & BANANA

Top 2 Ryvitas® (Pumpkin Seeds & Oats or Sunflower Seeds & Oats) with 1 tablespoon of natural peanut butter and 1 small sliced banana.

**NUTRITIONAL ANALYSIS PER SERVING**

225 calories; Total fat 8 g; Saturated fat 1 g; Protein 7 g; Carbohydrates 29 g; Fiber 6 g; Sodium 96 mg; Iron 1.2 mg; Calcium 21 mg; Folate 65 mcg; ALA 50 mg; Long-chain omega-3 0 mg

# The Low GI Eating Plan optimum weight gain chart

You are welcome to photocopy the chart on the following two pages and place it on the fridge (or a similar spot) for easy access. There is also a PDF version available for download from glycemicindex.com.

# THE LOW GI EATING PLAN OPTIMUM WEIGHT GAIN CHART

| | DATE | CURRENT WEIGHT IN POUNDS | WEIGHT CHANGE IN POUNDS | TOTAL WEIGHT GAIN SO FAR IN POUNDS |
|---|---|---|---|---|
| EXAMPLE | | | | |
| Pre-pregnancy | 1 May | 165 | - | - |
| Week 12 | 8 May | 165.5 | 0.5 | 0.5 |
| Week 13 | 15 May | 166 | 0.5 | 1 |
| Week 14 | 21 May | 167 | 1 | 2 |
| And so on | | | | |
| YOUR PREGNANCY | CURRENT DATE | CURRENT WEIGHT | WEIGHT CHANGE | TOTAL WEIGHT GAIN SO FAR |
| Pre-pregnancy | | | | |
| Week 1 | | | | |
| Week 2 | | | | |
| Week 3 | | | | |
| Week 4 | | | | |
| Week 5 | | | | |
| Week 6 | | | | |
| Week 7 | | | | |
| Week 8 | | | | |
| Week 9 | | | | |
| Week 10 | | | | |
| Week 11 | | | | |
| Week 12 | | | | |
| Week 13 | | | | |
| Week 14 | | | | |
| Week 15 | | | | |
| Week 16 | | | | |

| | | | | |
|---|---|---|---|---|
| Week 17 | | | | |
| Week 18 | | | | |
| Week 19 | | | | |
| Week 20 | | | | |
| Week 21 | | | | |
| Week 22 | | | | |
| Week 23 | | | | |
| Week 24 | | | | |
| Week 25 | | | | |
| Week 26 | | | | |
| Week 27 | | | | |
| Week 28 | | | | |
| Week 29 | | | | |
| Week 30 | | | | |
| Week 31 | | | | |
| Week 32 | | | | |
| Week 33 | | | | |
| Week 34 | | | | |
| Week 35 | | | | |
| Week 36 | | | | |
| Week 37 | | | | |
| Week 38 | | | | |
| Week 39 | | | | |
| Week 40 | Due date here | | | Your optimum range here |

# Resources and further information

## BABY, CHILD AND FAMILY HEALTH

### HEALTHYCHILDREN.ORG

healthychildren.org

This parenting website from the American Academy of Pediatrics offers everything from general information related to child health to more specific guidance on parenting issues. You'll also find information regarding the American Academy of Pediatrics' many programs and activities, their policies and guidelines, their publications and other child health resources.

### CHILDREN, YOUTH, AND FAMILIES EDUCATION AND RESEARCH NETWORK (CYFERNET)

www.cyfernet.org

CYFERnet provides high quality, research-based children and families resources culled from some of the best universities in the United States. It also has a database to help you identify local experts for children, youth and families should you need further help.

### SAFE KIDS USA

www.safekids.org

Provides important tips on keeping kids safe at home, on the playground, on the roads, and around water, with guidelines for different ages and stages.

## MATERNAL AND CHILD HEALTH BUREAU (MCHB)

mchb.hrsa.gov

A government program run by the U.S. Health and Human Services Department, the MCHB is committed to ensuring the health and well-being of every woman, infant and child in the United States. The site has a search function that allows you to find your state's MCHB contact information and connect you with local resources.

# BREASTFEEDING

## LA LECHE LEAGUE INTERNATIONAL

www.llli.org

Provides helpful information and mother-to-mother support through La Leche League's network of lay leaders and professional experts. In addition to attending local meetings, any new mother may call a local leader for assistance, contact a national breastfeeding hotline, e-mail the national office for help, search LLLI's database of research articles, visit the Ask the Experts columns or join an online computer chat for answers to her breastfeeding questions.

## INTERNATIONAL LACTATION CONSULTANTS ASSOCIATION

www.ilca.org

Enables you to search by state for a licensed lactation consultant near you to help with breastfeeding.

# FOOD SAFETY

## U.S. FOOD AND DRUG ADMINISTRATION

www.fda.gov/food/resourcesforyou/healtheducators/ucm081785.htm
The FDA Food Information Line: 1-888-SAFEFOOD
The Food Safety for Moms-to-Be page provides detailed information on food safety and nutrition issues during pregnancy, including advice on caffeine, mercury in fish, listeria, folate and iodine.

# GESTATIONAL DIABETES

## AMERICAN DIABETES ASSOCIATION (ADA)

www.diabetes.org

The ADA provides information and support for people living with diabetes, including women with gestational diabetes. Visit the page for your local ADA office to find out more about the services and support available to you.

## MEDICINES AND DRUGS

### ORGANIZATION OF TERATOLOGY INFORMATION SPECIALISTS (OTIS)

www.otispregnancy.org

OTIS Counselor Helpline: 866-626-6847

OTIS is a nonprofit organization made up of individual services (TIS) throughout North America. The organization is dedicated to providing accurate evidence-based, clinical information to patients and health-care professionals about medication exposures during pregnancy and lactation. The website offers a link to locate a service near you.

## MULTIPLE BIRTHS

### MEDLINE PLUS

www.nlm.nih.gov/medlineplus/twinstripletsmultiplebirths.html

This site, run by the National Institutes of Health (NIH), has valuable information and resources for parents expecting twins, triplets or more.

## NUTRITION AND HEALTHY EATING

### FOOD AND NUTRITION INFORMATION CENTER

United States Department of Agriculture National Agricultural Library

fnic.nal.usda.gov/lifecycle-nutrition/pregnancy

To speak to a Nutrition Information Specialist: 301-504-5414

This site provides women with the information they need to make good dietary choices during pregnancy and breastfeeding. Its staff of experienced registered dietitians is available Monday through Friday, 8:30 AM to 4:30 PM, to answer questions and help you locate resources.

### ACADEMY OF NUTRITION AND DIETETICS

www.eatright.org

This site provides nutritional information for infants and toddlers, and provides a link to help you locate registered dietitians in your area.

## POLYCYSTIC OVARY SYNDROME (PCOS)

### POLYCYSTIC OVARIAN SYNDROME ASSOCIATION (PCOSUPPORT)

www.pcosupport.org

PCOSupport is one of the leading support and advocacy groups for women with PCOS in the United States. Their website contains plenty of information on PCOS, including symptoms, diagnosis and treatment. Their community forums are also very helpful.

### PCOS CHALLENGE

www.pcoschallenge.com
One of the largest and most active support organizations for women with PCOS, PCOS Challenge offers an abundance of information on the condition on their website as well as online and offline support groups.

### SOULCYSTERS

www.soulcysters.com
Started in 2000 due to the lack of online information about PCOS, Soulcysters has become the largest online community for women with the condition. If you're looking for online support from fellow sufferers, this is the site to visit.

## POSTPARTUM DEPRESSION

### POSTPARTUM SUPPORT INTERNATIONAL (PSI)

www.postpartum.net
Help Line: 800-944-4PPD
Postpartum Support International is dedicated to helping women suffering from perinatal mood and anxiety disorders, including postpartum depression, the most common complication of childbirth. They also work to educate family, friends and health-care providers, so that moms and moms-to-be can get the support they need to recover. They host free live phone sessions every week with a PPD expert and can link you to local resources for recovery.

### MEDEDPPD.ORG

mededppd.org
This site was developed with the support of the National Institute of Mental Health (NIMH) to provide education about postpartum depression. Here, you can listen to the experiences of other mothers, get answers to your questions from experts in the field and find a health-care provider in your area trained in recognizing and treating PPD.

## PREGNANCY AND BIRTH

### AMERICAN PREGNANCY ASSOCIATION

www.americanpregnancy.org
The American Pregnancy Association is a national health organization committed to promoting reproductive and pregnancy wellness through education, research, advocacy and community awareness. Here, you can access a range of general health information on all topics related to pregnancy, giving birth, and breastfeeding.

## BABYCENTER

www.babycenter.com

The number one pregnancy and parenting web destination worldwide, BabyCenter provides moms with trusted advice from experts around the globe, friendship with other moms and support for every stage of pregnancy and child development.

# PREMATURE BIRTH

## PREEMIEHELP.COM

preemiehelp.com

Preemiehelp.com is an extensive resource for premature birth created by experts ranging from neuropsychologists to NICU nurses, caregivers to teachers. It provides information, community and solutions for parents of prematurely born babies and preemies themselves.

# SUDDEN INFANT DEATH SYNDROME (SIDS)

## NATIONAL SIDS RESOURCE CENTER

sidscenter.org

Provides information on reducing the risk of SIDS as well as support for those who have lost a child to SIDS or stillbirth.

# References

**CHAPTER 1: OPTIMIZING YOUR HEALTH AND LIFESTYLE**

Catalano, P. M., et al. "Fetuses of Obese Mothers Develop Insulin Resistance in Utero." *Diabetes Care* 32, no. 6 (2009): 1076–80.

Harizopoulou, V. C., et al. "Maternal Physical Activity Before and During Early Pregnancy as a Risk Factor for Gestational Diabetes Mellitus." *Acta Diabetologica* 47, Suppl. 1 (2010): 83–89. Published online July 18, 2009, doi: 10.1007/s00592-009-0136-1.

Hillemeier, M. M., et al. "Transition to Overweight or Obesity Among Women of Reproductive Age." *Journal of Women's Health* 20, no. 5 (2011): 703–10. Published online April 5, 2011, doi: 10.1089/jwh.2010.2397.

Ji, B. T., et al. "Paternal Cigarette Smoking and the Risk of Childhood Cancer Among Offspring of Nonsmoking Mothers." *Journal of the National Cancer Institute* 89, no. 3 (1997): 238–44.

Moran, L. J., et al. "Lifestyle Changes in Women with Polycystic Ovary Syndrome." *Cochrane Database of Systematic Review* 16, no. 2 (2011): CD007506. doi: 10.1002/14651858.CD007506.

National Library of Medicine. "Caffeine in the Diet." MedlinePlus. Last modified May 5, 2011, http://www.nlm.nih.gov/medlineplus/ency/article/002445.htm.

Schoeters, G. E., et al. "Biomonitoring and Biomarkers to Unravel the Risks from Prenatal Environmental Exposures for Later Health Outcomes." *The American Journal of Clinical Nutrition* 96, no. 6 Suppl (2011): 1964S–69S.

Wigle, D. T., et al. "Epidemiologic Evidence of Relationships Between Reproductive and Child Health Outcomes and Environmental Chemical Contaminants." *Journal of Toxicology and Environmental Health Part B: Critical Reviews* 11, no. 5–6 (2008): 373–517.

## CHAPTER 2: FERTILITY FOOD

American Thyroid Association. "Iodine Deficiency." Last modified June 4, 2012, http://www.thyroid.org/iodine-deficiency.

Chavarro, J. E., et al. "Diet and Lifestyle in the Prevention of Ovulatory Disorder Infertility." *Obstetrics and Gynecology* 110, no. 5 (2007): 1050–58.

———. "Dietary Fatty Acid Intakes and the Risk of Ovulatory Infertility." *The American Journal of Clinical Nutrition* 85, no. 1 (2007): 231–37.

Fung, T. T., et al. "Dietary Patterns, Meat Intake, and the Risk of Type 2 Diabetes in Women." *Archives of Internal Medicine* 164, no. 20 (2004): 2235–40.

Kramer, M. S., and R. Kakuma. "Energy and Protein Intake in Pregnancy." *Cochrane Database of Systematic Review* 2003, no. 4, doi: 10.1002/14651858.CD000032.

Lumley, J., et al. "Periconceptional Supplementation with Folate and/or Multivitamins for Preventing Neural Tube Defects." *Cochrane Database of Systematic Review* 2001, no. 3, doi: 10.1002/14651858.CD001056.

National Health and Medical Research Council Public Statement. "Iodine Supplementation for Pregnant and Breastfeeding Women." 2010, http://www.nhmrc.gov.au/publications/synopses/new45_syn.htm.

O'Connor, A. "Blood Levels of Trans Fats Are Declining in Americans." *New York Times*, February 8, 2012. http://well.blogs.nytimes.com/2012/02/08/blood-levels-of-trans-fats-are-declining-in-americans/.

Qiu, C., et al. "Risk of Gestational Diabetes Mellitus in Relation to Maternal Egg and Cholesterol Intake." *American Journal of Epidemiology* 173, no. 6 (2011): 649–58. Published online February 15, 2011, doi: 10.1093/aje/kwq425Epub.

Schulze, M. B., et al. "Processed Meat Intake and Incidence of Type 2 Diabetes in Younger and Middle-Aged Women." *Diabetologia* 46, no. 11 (2003): 1465–73.

Showell, M. G., et al. "Antioxidants for Male Subfertility." *Cochrane Database of Systematic Review* 2011, no. 1, doi: 10.1002/14651858.CD007411.pub2.

Song, Y., et al. "A Prospective Study of Red Meat Consumption and Type 2 Diabetes in Middle-Aged and Elderly Women: The Women's Health Study." *Diabetes Care* 27, no. 9 (2004): 2108–15.

The Mayo Clinic. "Pregnancy and Fish: What's Safe to Eat?" Published February 26, 2011, http://www.mayoclinic.com/health/pregnancy-and-fish/PR00158.

The Royal Women's Hospital. "Herbal Preparations in Pregnancy." [cited May, 2011]; http://www.thewomens.org.au /Herbalpreparationsinpregnancy.

Vang, A., et al. "Meats, Processed Meats, Obesity, Weight Gain and Occurrence of Diabetes among Adults: Findings from Adventist Health Studies." *Annals of Nutrition and Metabolism* 52, no. 2 (2008): 96–104. Published online March 18, 2008, doi: 10.1159/000121365.

Vesper, H. W., et al. "Levels of Plasma trans-Fatty Acids in Non-Hispanic White Adults in the United States in 2000 and 2009." *The Journal of the American Medical Association* 307, no. 6 (2012): 562–63.

Zhang, C., et al. "A Prospective Study of Dietary Patterns, Meat Intake and the Risk of Gestational Diabetes Mellitus." *Diabetologia* 49, no. 11 (2006): 2604–13.

## CHAPTER 3: THE BEST CONCEIVABLE DIET FOR PREGNANCY

Adgent, M.A. "Environmental Tobacco Smoke and Sudden Infant Death Syndrome: A Review." *Birth Defects Research Part B: Developmental and Reproductive Toxicology* 77, no. 1 (2006): 69–85.

Burks, A. W., et al. "ICON Guidelines for Food Allergy." *The Journal of Allergy and Clinical Immunology* 129, no. 5 (2012): 906–92. Excerpt available from: American Academy of Allergy, Asthma & Immunology, www .aaaai.org/ask-the-expert/dietary-intervention-during-pregnancy.aspx.

Crozier, T. W. M., et al. "Espresso Coffees, Caffeine and Chlorogenic Acid Intake: Potential Health Implications." *Food and Function* 3, no. 1 (2012): 30–33. Published online November 30, 2011, doi: 10.1039 /C1FO10240K.

Czeizel, A. E. "Periconceptional Folic Acid and Multivitamin Supplementation for the Prevention of Neural Tube Defects and Other Congenital Abnormalities." *Birth Defects Research Part A: Clinical and Molecular Teratology* 85, no. 4 (2009): 260–68.

Desbrow, B., et al. "An Examination of Consumer Exposure to Caffeine from Retail Coffee Outlets." *Food and Chemical Toxicology* 45, no. 9 (2007): 1588–92.

Donahue, S. M, et al. "Prenatal Fatty Acid Status and Child Adiposity at Age 3 Y: Results from a US Pregnancy Cohort." *The American Journal of Clinical Nutrition* 93, no. 4 (2011): 780–88. Published online February 10, 2011, doi: 10.3945/ajcn.110.005801.

Fleith, M., and M. T. Clandinin. "Dietary PUFA for Preterm and Term Infants: Review of Clinical Studies." *Critical Reviews in Food Science and Nutrition* 45, no. 3 (2005): 205–29.

Fraser, R. B., et al. "Insulin Sensitivity in Third Trimester Pregnancy. A randomized study of dietary effects." *British Journal of Obstetrics and Gynaecology* 95, no. 3 (1988): 223–29.

Food Standards Australia New Zealand. "Mercury in Fish." Last modified September 2011, http://www.foodstandards.gov.au/foodmatters/mercuryinfish.cfm.

Gibson, R. A., et al. "Conversion of Linoleic Acid and Alpha-Linolenic Acid to Long-Chain Polyunsaturated Fatty Acids (Lcpufas), with a Focus on Pregnancy, Lactation and the First 2 Years of Life." *Maternal & Child Nutrition* 7, Suppl 2 (2011): 17–26. Published online March 2, 2011, doi: 10.1111/j.1740-8709.2011.00299.

Gluckman, P. D., et al. "Effect of In Utero and Early-Life Conditions on Adult Health and Disease." *New England Journal of Medicine* 359, no. 1 (2008): 61–73.

Godfrey, K. M., et al. "Epigenetic Gene Promoter Methylation at Birth is Associated with Child's Later Adiposity." *Diabetes* 60, no. 5 (2011): 1528–34.

Goh, Y.I., et al. "Prenatal Multivitamin Supplementation and Rates of Congenital Anomalies: A Meta-Analysis." *Journal of Obstetrics and Gynaecology Canada* 28, no. 8 (2006): 680–89.

Klebanoff, M. A., et al. "Fish Consumption, Erythrocyte Fatty Acids, and Preterm Birth." *Obstetrics and Gynecology* 117, no. 5 (2011): 1071–77. doi: 10.1097/AOG.0b013e31821645dc.

Larque, E., et al. "Perinatal Supply and Metabolism of Long-Chain Polyunsaturated Fatty Acids: Importance for the Early Development of the Nervous System." *Annals of the New York Academy of Sciences* 967 (2002): 299–310.

Lau, S. L., et al. "Serum 25-Hydroxyvitamin D and Glycated Haemoglobin Levels in Women with Gestational Diabetes Mellitus." *Medical Journal of Australia* 194, no. 7 (2011): 334–37.

Linnet, K. M., et al. "Maternal Lifestyle Factors in Pregnancy Risk of Attention Deficit Hyperactivity Disorder and Associated Behaviors: Review of the Current Evidence." *The American Journal of Psychiatry* 160, no. 6 (2003): 1028–40.

McGowan, C.A., and F. M. McAuliffe. "The Influence of Maternal Glycaemia and Dietary Glycaemic Index on Pregnancy Outcomes in Healthy Mothers." *British Journal of Nutrition* 104, no. 2 (2010): 153–59.

Monasta L., et al. "Early-Life Determinants of Overweight and Obesity: A Review of Systematic Reviews." *Obesity Reviews* 11, no. 10 (2010): 695–708. doi: 10.1111/j.1467-789X.2010.00735.x.

Moses, R. G., and J. C. Brand-Miller. "The Use of a Low Glycemic Index Diet in Pregnancy: An Evolving Treatment Paradigm." *Diabetes Research and Clinical Practice* 91, no. 1 (2011): 13–14.

National Health and Medical Research Council Public Statement. "Iodine Supplementation for Pregnant and Breastfeeding Women." 2010, http://www.nhmrc.gov.au/publications/synopses/new45_syn.htm.

Office of Dietary Supplements, National Institute of Health. "Dietary Supplement Fact Sheet: Vitamin D." Accessed June 24, 2011. http://ods .od.nih.gov/factsheets/vitaminD-HealthProfessional/.

———. "Dietary Supplement Fact Sheet: Folate." Accessed April 15, 2009. http://ods.od.nih.gov/factsheets/Folate-HealthProfessional/.

Rhodes, E.R., et al. "Effects of a Low Glycemic Index Diet in Overweight and Obese Pregnant Women: A Pilot Randomized Controlled Trial." *The American Journal of Clinical Nutrition* 92, no. 6 (2010): 1306–15.

Salmasi, G., et al. "Environmental Tobacco Smoke Exposure and Perinatal Outcomes: A Systematic Review and Meta-Analyses." *Acta Obstetricia et Gynecologica Scandinavica* 89, no. 4 (2010): 423–41.

Sandovici, I., et al. "Maternal Diet and Aging Alter the Epigenetic Control of a Promoter-Enhancer Interaction at the Hnf4a Gene in Rat Pancreatic Islets." *Proceedings of the National Academy of Sciences of the United States of America* 108, no. 13 (2011): 5449–54. Published online March 8, 2011, doi: 10.1073/pnas.1019007108.

The Australasian Society of Clinical Immunology and Allergy. "Allergy Prevention in Children 2010." [cited May, 2011] http://www.allergy.org .au/content/view/182/127/.

The Royal Women's Hospital. "Herbal Preparations in Pregnancy." [cited May, 2011] http://www.thewomens.org.au /Herbalpreparationsinpregnancy.

## CHAPTER 4: IDEAL WEIGHT GAIN

Bevier, W., and L. Jovanovic. "Weight Gain and Gestational Diabetes Mellitus Is a Sensitive Issue." *Diabetes Care* 31, no. 1 (2008): e1.

Callaway, L. K., et al. "The Prevalence and Impact of Overweight and Obesity in Australian Obstetric Population." *Medical Journal of Australia* 184, no. 2 (2006): 56–59.

Crozier, S. R., et al. "Weight Gain in Pregnancy and Childhood Body Composition: Findings from the Southampton Women's Survey." *The American Journal of Clinical Nutrition* 91, no. 6 (2010): 1745–51.

Fraser A., et al. "Associations of Gestational Weight Gain with Maternal Body Mass Index, Waist Circumference, and Blood Pressure Measured 16 Y after Pregnancy: The Avon Longitudinal Study of Parents and Children (ALSPAC)." *The American Journal of Clinical Nutrition* 93, no. 6 (2011): 1285–92.

Gardner, B., et al. "Changing Diet and Physical Activity to Reduce Gestational Weight Gain: A Meta-Analysis." *Obesity Reviews* 12, no. 7 (2011): E602–20.

Godfrey, K. M., et al. "Epigenetic Gene Promoter Methylation at Birth is Associated with Child's Later Adiposity." *Diabetes* 60, no. 5 (2011): 1528–34.

Jeffries K., et al. "Reducing Excessive Weight Gain in Pregnancy: A Randomized Controlled Trial." *Medical Journal of Australia* 191, no. 8 (2009): 429–33.

Kinnunen, T. I., et al. "Preventing Excessive Weight Gain During Pregnancy—A Controlled Trial in Primary Health Care." *European Journal of Clinical Nutrition* 61, no. 7 (2007): 884–91.

Larsen, T. M., et al. "Diets with High or Low Protein Content and Glycemic Index for Weight-Loss Maintenance." *New England Journal of Medicine.* 363, no. 22 (2010): 2102–13.

Lawlor, D. A., et al. "Does Maternal Weight Gain in Pregnancy Have Long-Term Effects on Offspring Adiposity? A Sibling Study in a Prospective Cohort of 146,894 Men from 136,050 Families." *The American Journal of Clinical Nutrition* 94, no. 1 (2011): 142–48.

Ludwig, D., and J. Currie. "The Association between Pregnancy Weight Gain and Birthweight: A Within-Family Comparison." *The Lancet* 376, no. 9745 (2010): 984–90.

McMillan-Price, J., et al. "Comparison of 4 Diets of Varying Glycemic Load on Weight Loss and Cardiovascular Risk Reduction in Overweight and Obese Young Adults: A Randomized Controlled Trial." *Archives Internal Medicine* 166, no. 14 (2006): 1466–75.

Oken, E., and M. W. Gillman. "Fetal Origins of Obesity." *Obesity Research* 11, no. 3 (2003): 496–506.

Skouteris, H., et al. "Prevention Excessive Gestational Weight Gain: A Systematic Review of Interventions." *Obesity Reviews* 11, no. 11 (2010): 757–68.

Siega-Riz, A-M., and B. Laraia. "The Implications of Maternal Overweight and Obesity on the Course of Pregnancy and Birth Outcomes." *Maternal Child Health Journal* 10, no. 5 Suppl (2006): S153–56.

Siega-Riz, A-M., et al. "A Systematic Review of Outcomes of Maternal Weight Gain According to the Institute Of Medicine Recommendations: Birth Weight, Fetal Growth, and Postpartum Weight Reduction." *American Journal of Obstetrics and Gynecology* 201, no. 4 (2009): 339.e1–14.

Thangaratinam, S., and K. Jolly. "Obesity in Pregnancy: A Review of Reviews on the Effectiveness of Interventions." *BJOG: An International Journal of Obstetrics & Gynaecology* 117, no. 11 (2010): 1309–12.

Wolff, S., et al. "A Randomized Trial of the Effects of Dietary Counseling on Gestational Weight Gain and Glucose Metabolism in Obese Pregnant Women." *International Journal of Obesity* 32, no. 3 (2008): 495–501.

Wrotniak, B. H., et al. "Gestational Weight Gain and Risk of Overweight in the Offspring at Age 7 in a Multicenter, Multiethnic Cohort Study." *The American Journal of Clinical Nutrition* 87, no. 6 (2008): 1818–24.

## CHAPTER 5: BLOOD GLUCOSE LEVELS IN PREGNANCY

Atkinson, F., et al. "International Tables of Glycemic Index and Glycemic Load Values: 2008." *Diabetes Care* 31, no. 12 (2008): 2281–83.

Bao, J., et al. "Prediction of Postprandial Glycemia and Insulinemia in Lean, Young, Healthy Adults: Glycemic Load Compared with Carbohydrate Content Alone." *The American Journal of Clinical Nutrition* 93, no. 5 (2011): 984–96.

Barclay, A., et al. "Glycemic Index, Glycemic Load and Chronic Disease Risk—A Meta-Analysis of Observational Studies." *The American Journal of Clinical Nutrition* 87, no. 3 (2008): 627–37.

Boden G. "Fuel Metabolism in Pregnancy and in Gestational Diabetes Mellitus." *Obstetrics & Gynecology Clinics of North America* 23, no. 1 (1996): 1–10.

Brand-Miller, J. C. "Glycemic Load and Chronic Disease." *Nutrition Reviews* 61 no. 5 Pt 2 (2003): S49–55.

———. "Postprandial Glycemica, Glycemic Index, and the Prevention of Type 2 Diabetes." *The American Journal of Clinical Nutrition* 80, no. 2 (2004): 243–44.

Brand-Miller, J. C., et al. "A New Food Labelling Program for the Glycemic Index." *Proceedings of the Nutrition Society of Australia* 25 (2001): S21.

Brand-Miller, J. C., et al. "Glycemic Index, Postprandial Glycemia, and the Shape of the Curve in Healthy Subjects: Analysis of a Database of More than 1000 Foods." *The American Journal of Clinical Nutrition* 89, no. 1 (2009): 97–105.

Brand-Miller, J. C., et al. "Physiological Validation of the Concept of Glycemic Load in Lean Young Adults." *The Journal of Nutrition* 133 no. 9 (2003): 2728–32.

Brand-Miller, J. C., et al. "Glycemic Index and Obesity." *The American Journal of Clinical Nutrition* 76, no. 1 (2002): 281S–5S.

Butte, N. F. "Carbohydrate and Lipid Metabolism in Pregnancy: Normal Compared with Gestational Diabetes Mellitus." *The American Journal of Clinical Nutrition* 71, no. 5 Suppl (2000): 1256S–61S.

Clapp III, J. F. "Effect of Dietary Carbohydrate on the Glucose and Insulin Response to Mixed Caloric Intake and Exercise in Both Nonpregnant and Pregnant Women." *Diabetes Care* 21, Suppl 2 (1998): 107–12.

Combs, C. A., et al. "Relationship of Fetal Macrosomia to Maternal Postprandial Glucose Control During Pregnancy." *Diabetes Care* 15, no. 10 (1992): 1251–57.

Deirerlein, A. L., et al. "The Association Between Maternal Glucose Concentration and Child BMI at Age 3 Years." *Diabetes Care* 34, no. 2 (2011): 480–84.

Fraser, R. B., et al. "Insulin Sensitivity in Third Trimester Pregnancy. A Randomized Study of Dietary Effects." *BJOG: An International Journal of Obstetrics & Gynaecology* 95, no. 3 (1988): 223–29.

Frost, G., and A. Dornhorst. "The Relevance of the Glycaemic Index to our Understanding of Dietary Carbohydrates." *Diabetic Medicine: A Journal of the British Diabetic Association* 17, no. 5 (2000): 336–45.

Gillen, L., et al. "The Type and Frequency of Consumption of Carbohydrate Rich Foods May Play a Role in the Clinical Expression of Insulin Resistance During Pregnancy." *Nutrition & Dietetics* 59, no. 2 (2002): 135–43.

Kaushik, S., et al. "Glycemic Index, Retinal Vascular Caliber, and Stroke Mortality." *Stroke: A Journal of Cerebral Circulation* 40, no. 1 (2009): 206–12.

Louie, J. C., et al. "Glycemic Index and Pregnancy: A Systematic Literature Review." *Journal of Nutrition and Metabolism* 2010: 282464 Published online January 2, 2011, doi: 10.1155/2010/282464.

Luo, Z. C., et al. "Maternal Glucose Tolerance in Pregnancy Affects Fetal Insulin Sensitivity." *Diabetes Care* 33, no. 9 (2010): 2055–61.

Metzger, B. E., et al. "Hyperglycemia and Adverse Pregnancy Outcomes." *New England Journal of Medicine* 358, no. 19 (2008): 1991–2002.

Moses, R. G., et al. "Effect of a Low-Glycemic-Index Diet During Pregnancy on Obstetric Outcomes." *The American Journal of Clinical Nutrition* 84, no. 4 (2006): 807–12.

Moses, R. G., et al. "Maternal Diet and Infant Size at 2 Y after the Completion of a Study of A Low Glycemic Index Diet in Pregnancy." *The American Journal of Clinical Nutrition* 86, no. 6 (2007): 1806.

Parretti, E., et al. "Sonographic Evaluation of Fetal Growth and Body Composition in Women with Different Degrees of Normal Glucose Metabolism." *Diabetes Care* 26, no. 10 (2003): 2741–48.

Radesky, J. S., et al. "Diet During Early Pregnancy and Development of Gestational Diabetes." *Paediatric and Perinatal Epidemiology* 22, no. 1 (2008): 47–59.

Scholl, T. O., et al. "Maternal Glucose Concentration Influences Fetal Growth, Gestation and Pregnancy Complications." *American Journal of Epidemiology* 154, no. 6 (2001): 514–20.

Shaw, G. M., et al. "Neural Tube Defects Associated with Maternal Periconceptional Dietary Intake of Simple Sugars and Glycemic Index." *The American Journal of Clinical Nutrition* 78, no. 5 (2003): 972–78.

Small, P., and J. Brand-Miller. "From Complex Carbohydrate to Glycemic Index: Tracing the Controversy." *Nutrition Today* 44, no. 6 (2009): 244–45. doi: 10.1097/NT.0b013e3181c5fcd5.

Tallarigo, L, et al. "Relation of Glucose Tolerance to Complications of Pregnancy in Nondiabetic Women." *New England Journal of Medicine* 315, no. 16 (1986): 989–92.

Wang, Y., et al. "Dietary Variables and Glucose Tolerance in Pregnancy." *Diabetes Care* 23, no. 4 (2000): 460–64.

Wei, J. N., et al. "Low Birth Weight and High Birth Weight Infants Are Both at an Increased Risk to Have Type 2 Diabetes among Schoolchildren in Taiwan." *Diabetes Care* 26, no. 2 (2003): 343–48.

Yazdy, M. M., et al. "Maternal Dietary Glycemic Intake and the Risk of Neural Tube Defects." *American Journal of Epidemiology* 171, no. 4 (2010): 407–14.

Yu, Z. B., et al. "Birth Weight and Subsequent Risk of Obesity: A Systematic Review and Meta-Analysis." *Obesity Reviews* 12, no. 7 (2011): 525–42.

Zhang, C., et al. "Dietary Fiber Intake, Dietary Glycemic Load, and the Risk for Gestational Diabetes Mellitus." *Diabetes Care* 29, no. 10 (2006): 2223–30.

**CHAPTER 6: EXERCISE IN PREGNANCY**

Artal, R., et al. "Guidelines of the American College of Obstetricians and Gynecologists for Exercise During Pregnancy and the Postpartum Period." *British Journal of Sports Medicine* 37, no. 1 (2003): 6–12.

Hopkins, S. A., et al. "Exercise Training in Pregnancy Reduces Offspring Size without Changes in Maternal Insulin Sensitivity." *The Journal of Clinical Endocrinology & Metabolism* 95, no. 5 (2010): 2080–88.

Sports Medicine Australia. "SMA Statement: The Benefits and Risks of Exercise During Pregnancy." *Journal of Science and Medicine in Sport* 5, no. 1 (2002): 11–19.

Thomas, D. E., et al. "Carbohydrate Feeding Before Exercise: Effect of Glycemic Index." *International Journal of Sports Medicine* 12, no. 2 (1991): 180–86.

Tobias, D. K., et al. "Physical Activity Before and During Pregnancy and Risk of Gestational Diabetes Mellitus: A Meta-Analysis." *Diabetes Care* 34, no. 1 (2011): 223–29. Published online September 27, 2010, doi: 10.2337 /dc10-1368.

Zavorsky, G. S., and L.D. Longo. "Adding Strength Training, Exercise Intensity, and Caloric Expenditure to Exercise Guidelines in Pregnancy." *Obstetrics and Gynecology* 117, no. 6 (2011): 1399–1402.

Zavorsky, G. S., and L.D. Longo. "Exercise Guidelines in Pregnancy: New Perspectives." *Sports Medicine* 41, no. 5 (2011): 345–60.

**CHAPTER 7: GESTATIONAL DIABETES: WHY SUCH A BIG DEAL?**

American Pregnancy Association. "Glucose Challenge Screening & Glucose Tolerance Test." Last updated August 2007, http://www .americanpregnancy.org/prenataltesting/glucosetest.html.

Boland, E., et al. "Limitations of Conventional Methods of Self-Monitoring of Blood Glucose: Lessons Learned From 3 Days 0f Continuous Glucose Sensing in Pediatric Patients with Type 1 Diabetes." *Diabetes Care* 24, no. 11 (2001): 1858–62.

Brand, J. C., et al. "Low-Glycemic Index Foods Improve Long-Term Glycemic Control in NIDDM." *Diabetes Care* 14, no. 2 (1991): 95–101.

Brand-Miller, J., et al. "Low-Glycemic Index Diets in the Management of Diabetes: A Meta-Analysis of Randomized Controlled Trials." *Diabetes Care* 26, no. 8 (2003): 2261–67.

Chen, L., et al. "Prospective Study of Pre-Gravid Sugar-Sweetened Beverage Consumption and the Risk of Gestational Diabetes Mellitus." *Diabetes Care* 32, no. 12 (2009): 756.

Crowther, C. A., et al. "Effect of Treatment of Gestational Diabetes Mellitus on Pregnancy Outcomes." *New England Journal of Medicine* 352, no. 24 (2005): 2477–86.

de Veciana M., et al. "Postprandial Versus Preprandial Blood Glucose Monitoring in Women with Gestational Diabetes Mellitus Requiring Insulin Therapy." *New England Journal of Medicine* 333, no. 19 (1995): 1237–41.

Eunice Kennedy Shriver National Institute of Child Health and Human Development. "What Should I Do if I Have Gestational Diabetes?" Last modified August 16, 2006, http://www.nichd.nih.gov /publications/pubs/gest_diabetes/sub4.cfm.

Gilbertson, H. R., et al. "The Effect of Flexible Low Glycemic Index Dietary Advice Versus Measured Carbohydrate Exchange Diets on Glycemic Control in Children with Type 1 Diabetes." *Diabetes Care* 24, no. 7 (2001): 1137–43.

Grant, S. M., et al. "Effect of a Low Glycaemic Index Diet on Blood Glucose in Women with Gestational Hyperglycaemia." *Diabetes Research and Clinical Practice* 91, no. 1 (2011): 15–22.

Landon, M. B., et al. "Neonatal Morbidity in Pregnancy Complicated by Diabetes Mellitus: Predictive Value of Maternal Glycemic Profiles." *American Journal of Obstetrics & Gynecology* 156, no. 5 (1987): 1089–95.

Louie, J. C., et al. "A Randomized Controlled Trial Investigating the Effects of a Low–Glycemic Index Diet on Pregnancy Outcomes in Gestational Diabetes Mellitus." *Diabetes Care* 34, no. 11 (2011): 2341–46.

Moses, R. G., et al. "Can a Low-Glycemic Index Diet Reduce the Need for Insulin in Gestational Diabetes Mellitus? A Randomized Trial." *Diabetes Care* 32, no. 6 (2009): 996–1000.

Moses, R. G., and D. Calvert. "Pregnancy Outcomes in Women without Gestational Diabetes Mellitus Related to the Maternal Glucose Level. Is There a Continuum of Risk?" *Diabetes Care* 18, no. 12 (1995): 1527–33.

Moses, R. G., et al. "The Incidence of Gestational Diabetes in the Illawarra Area of New Wales." *Australian and New Zealand Journal of Obstetrics and Gynaecology* 34, no. 4 (1994): 425–27.

Moses, R. G., et al. "Gestational Diabetes Mellitus. At What Time Should the Postprandial Glucose Level Be Monitored?" *Australian and New Zealand Journal of Obstetrics and Gynaecology* 39, no. 4 (1999): 458–60.

Pettitt, D. J., et al. "Excessive Obesity in Offspring of Pima Indian Women with Diabetes During Pregnancy." *New England Journal of Medicine* 308, no. 5 (1983): 242–45.

Retnakaran, R. "Glucose Intolerance in Pregnancy and Future Risk of Pre-Diabetes or Diabetes." *Diabetes Care* 31, no. 10 (2008): 2026–31.

Sermer, M., et al. "Impact of Increasing Carbohydrate Intolerance on Maternal-Fetal Outcomes In 3637 Women Without Gestational Diabetes." *American Journal of Obstetrics & Gynecology* 173, no. 1 (1995): 146–56.

Slama, G. "Clinical Significance of Post-Prandial Blood Glucose Excursions in Type 1 and Type 2 Diabetes Mellitus." *International Journal of Clinical Practice* 112 Suppl (2000): 9–12.

Thorburn, A., et al. "Slowly Digested and Absorbed Carbohydrate in Traditional Bushfoods: A Protective Factor Against Diabetes?" *The American Journal of Clinical Nutrition* 45, no. 1 (1987): 98–106.

Tieu, J., et al. "Dietary Advice in Pregnancy for Preventing Gestational Diabetes Mellitus." *Cochrane Database of Systematic Review* 16, no. 2 (2008): CD006674. doi: 10.1002/14651858.CD006674.pub2.

## CHAPTER 8: LACTATION AND LOOKING AFTER YOURSELF

Liston, J. "Breastfeeding and the Use of Recreational Drugs—Alcohol, Caffeine, Nicotine and Marijuana." *Breastfeeding Review: Australian Breastfeeding Association* 6, no. 2 (1998): 27–30.

Growing Up in Australia. "The Longitudinal Study of Australian Children: Annual Report 2006–2007." http://www.growingupinaustralia.gov.au/pubs/ar/ar200607/breastfeeding.html.

Ip, S., et al. "Breastfeeding and Maternal and Infant Health Outcomes in Developed Countries." United States Agency for Healthcare Research and Quality Evidence Report/Technology Assessment 153 (2007): 1–186.

Ip, S., et al. "A Summary of the Agency for Healthcare Research and Quality's Evidence Report on Breast-Feeding in Developed Countries." *Breastfeeding Medicine: The Official Journal of the Academy of Breastfeeding Medicine* 4, Suppl 1 (2009): S17–30.

Hauck, F. R., et al. "Breastfeeding and Reduced Risk of Sudden Infant Death Syndrome: A Meta-analysis." *Pediatrics* 128, no. 1 (2011): 103–10.

Gouveri, E., et al. "Breastfeeding and Diabetes." *Current Diabetes Reviews* 7, no. 2 (2011): 135–42.

Kramer, M. S. "Breastfeeding, Complementary (Solid) Foods, and Long-Term Risk of Obesity." *The American Journal of Clinical Nutrition* 91, no. 3 (2010): 500–501.

Prescott, S. L., and M. L. Tang. "The Australasian Society of Clinical Immunology and Allergy Position Statement: Summary of Allergy

Prevention in Children." *Medical Journal of Australia* 182, no. 9 (2005): 464–67.

Taylor, J. S., et al. "A Systematic Review of the Literature Associating Breastfeeding With Type 2 Diabetes and Gestational Diabetes." *Journal of the American College of Nutrition* 24, no. 5 (2005): 320–26.

Wong, S., et al. "Substance Use in Pregnancy." *Journal of Obstetrics and Gynaecology Canada* 33, no. 4 (2011): 367–84.

## CHAPTER 9: WEANING YOUR BABY

Greer, F. R., et al. "Effects of Early Nutritional Interventions on the Development of Atopic Disease in Infants and Children: The Role of Maternal Dietary Restriction, Breastfeeding, Timing of Introduction of Complementary Foods, and Hydrolyzed Formulas." *Pediatrics* 121, no. 1 (2008): 183–91.

Prescott, S. L., and M. L. Tang. "The Australasian Society of Clinical Immunology and Allergy Position Statement: Summary of Allergy Prevention in Children." *Medical Journal of Australia* 182, no. 9 (2005): 464–67.

The Australasian Society of Clinical Immunology and Allergy. "Allergy Prevention in Children 2010." [cited May, 2011] http://www.allergy.org.au/content/view/182/127/.

## CHAPTER 10: THE LOW GI EATING PLAN—PUTTING IT INTO ACTION

Huang, C. J., et al. "Associations of Breakfast Skipping with Obesity and Health-Related Quality of Life: Evidence From a National Survey in Taiwan." *International Journal of Obesity* 34, no. 4 (2010): 720–25. Published online January 12, 2010, doi: 10.1038/ijo.2009.285.

Institute of Medicine (US) and National Research Council (US) Committee to Reexamine IOM Pregnancy Weight Guidelines. *Weight Gain During Pregnancy: Reexamining the Guidelines.* Washington, DC: 2009.

Koh-Banerjee, P., et al. "Changes in Whole-Grain, Bran, and Cereal Fiber Consumption in Relation to 8-Y Weight Gain Among Men." *The American Journal of Clinical Nutrition* 80, no. 5 (2004): 1237–45.

Kramer, M. S., and R. Kakuma. "Energy and Protein Intake in Pregnancy." *Cochrane Database of Systematic Review* 2003, no. 4, doi: 10.1002/14651858.CD000032.

Liu, S., et al. "Relation Between Changes in Intakes of Dietary Fiber and Grain Products and Changes in Weight and Development of Obesity among

Middle-Aged Women." *The American Journal of Clinical Nutrition* 78, no. 5 (2003): 920–27.

Mizutani, T., et al. "Association of Maternal Lifestyles Including Smoking During Pregnancy with Childhood Obesity." *Obesity* 15, no. 12 (2007): 3133–39.

Qiu, C., et al. "Risk of Gestational Diabetes Mellitus in Relation to Maternal Egg and Cholesterol Intake." *American Journal of Epidemiology* 173, no. 6 (2011): 649–58. Published online February 15, 2011, doi: 10.1093/aje /kwq425Epub.

Rampersaud, G. C., et al. "Breakfast Habits, Nutritional Status, Body Weight, and Academic Performance in Children and Adolescents." *Journal of the American Dietetic Association* 105, no. 5 (2005): 743–60; quiz 761–62.

Smith, K. J., et al. "Skipping Breakfast: Longitudinal Associations with Cardiometabolic Risk Factors in the Childhood Determinants of Adult Health Study." *The American Journal of Clinical Nutrition* 92, no. 6 (2010): 1316–25. Published online October 6, 2010, doi: 10.3945 /ajcn.2010.30101.

Parrott, S. M., et al. "Maternal Cereal Consumption and Adequacy of Micronutrient Intake in the Periconceptional Period." *Public Health Nutrition* 12, no. 8 (2009): 1276–83. Published online November 10, 2008, doi: 10.1017/S136898000800388.

Zhang, C., et al. "A Prospective Study of Dietary Patterns, Meat Intake and the Risk of Gestational Diabetes Mellitus." *Diabetologia* 49, no. 11 (2006): 2604–13.

## CHAPTER 13: TOP PREGNANCY SUPER FOODS

American Pregnancy Association. "Nutrient Guidelines." Last updated October 2008, http://www.americanpregnancy.org/pregnancyhealth /nutrientguidelines.htm.

Office of Dietary Supplements, National Institute of Health. "Dietary Supplement Fact Sheet: Iodine." Accessed June 2011. http://ods.od.nih .gov/factsheets/iodine-QuickFacts..

# Acknowledgments

*The Low GI Eating Plan for an Optimal Pregnancy* has had a very long gestation and many individuals have contributed to a successful delivery. The seed was planted in 2004 when we began the first study applying a low GI diet to healthy pregnancies. The study was undertaken at Wollongong Hospital with the skills and expertise of research dietitians Professor Linda Tapsell and Ms. Megan Luebke, and the collaboration of private practice obstetricians Dr. W. Davis and Dr. K. Coleman.

A second study, this time in women with gestational diabetes, began in 2008 at Royal Prince Alfred Hospital in Sydney, with a team of individuals including endocrinologists Tania Markovic and Glynis Ross; accredited practicing dietitians Jimmy Louie (who also undertook his PhD), Deborah Foote and Natasha Davis; endocrinology registrar Nimalie Perera; and the willing assistance of Professor Jon Hyett, Head of Obstetrics, and Professor Dennis Yue, Head of Diabetes at RPAH.

Two studies, both in healthy pregnancies, are continuing: one in Sydney (with project funding from the National Health and Medical Research Council of Australia and the University of Sydney) and one in Wollongong with additional involvement of dietitians Shelly Charters, Dawn Tan and Ruth Hart, and PhD student Nathalie Kizirian.

Over the same time frame, we also undertook the first controlled trial of a low GI diet in women with polycystic ovary syndrome (PCOS), a condition often diagnosed in women who have difficulty conceiving. Endocrinologist Dr. Warren Kidson conceived the original idea, and Professor Kate Steinbeck, then Head of Metabolism and Obesity Services at Royal Prince Alfred Hospital (and now Medical Foundation

Chair of Adolescent Medicine at University of Sydney), oversaw the clinical aspects.

The idea of a lay book devoted to pregnancy grew naturally out of these studies. Our literary agent, Philippa Sandall, clinched the deal, and encouraged our efforts, identifying media releases and newspaper headlines, and otherwise stoking the fires of enthusiasm. In early 2011, we began the long process of distilling the scientific knowledge into a coherent form suitable for the general reader.

We are grateful to many individuals who provided valuable comments and suggestions on the manuscript: Philippa Sandall; John Miller; Lee Dixon; exercise specialists Margaret Torode and Susan White; home economist Alison Roberts, who devised and tested the majority of the recipes; and the friends and family who bravely tested the remaining recipes: Janice Windsor, Rhiannon Brazier, Katie Dodd, and Lee and Colin Dixon. Miriam Chin and Kathleen Richardson helped us with the nutrient analysis of the recipes.

Of course, there would be no book without a publisher. We remain eternally grateful to Fiona Hazard of Hachette Australia, our editor, Kate Ballard, and sales and marketing staff.

For our North American edition, we owe a big thank you to our publisher Matthew Lore and our editor Cara Bedick, as well as Molly Cavanaugh, Jack Palmer and recipe modifier Sue McCloskey Fisher.

We thank each and every one of you, with a big hug and a warm smile, with the sure knowledge that all our efforts will make a contribution to improving the health of a future generation of mothers and babies.

# Index

salt
  in canned goods, 194
  in diet, 26, 46, 147
  in processed foods, 144,
    195, 196
sardines, canned, 194
saturated fats, 167–68
  father's diet high in, 14
  and gestational diabetes,
    103, 115
  and intrauterine
    programming, 101
  in processed foods, 111,
    167, 169
  sources of, 169, 199
sauces, 195
Scholl, Theresa, 79
seafood, 43, 44, 46–47, 164
  and food safety, 31, 50
  iodine in, 26
  mercury in, 26–27, 53–54
  protein in, 164
seaweed supplements, caution
  about, 32, 46, 47
seeds. See nuts and seeds
servings
  of caffeine, 17, 52
  of calcium-rich foods,
    44–45
  of carbohydrates, 109–10
  of fish, 26–27, 53–54
  of low nutrient density
    foods, 158–59
  of nutrient-dense foods,
    156–58, 173–74
  plate model for, 161–62,
    189–90
sexually transmitted diseases
  (STDs), 18
shopping for low GI foods,
    202
  GI symbol, 188, 203
  in place of high GI foods,
    174–75
SIDS (sudden infant death
  syndrome), 15, 55, 132,
    301
"6 out of 7" rule, 112
small babies (less than 5
  pounds, 8 ounces)
  and blood glucose level
    during gestation, 75–76
  complications in early
    months of life, 79
  and exercise of mother,
    83
  and food supplements, 27,
    68, 76
  and mother's weight gain
    during pregnancy, 62

special care for, 135–36
smoking
  avoiding during pregnancy,
    54–55
  and breastfeeding, 132
  quitting pre-pregnancy, 15
smoothies and milkshakes,
    180. See also fruit
    smoothies
snacks, 161, 188–89
  for breastfeeding, 129–30
  summer menu ideas, 210–11
  winter menu ideas, 212–13
soft drinks, avoiding, 29, 30,
    52, 159
solid foods for baby, 144–47
soluble fiber, 78
"sometimes" foods, 147. See
    also weaning
soups for babies, 146
Southampton Women's Study
  (UK), 63
soy products, 164, 165, 201
  nutrient density of, 157–58
  as source of fluids, 179–80
sperm quality, 14, 33
spices, 197
spina bifida, 80–81
Starbucks, 178
starch, 78
STDs (sexually transmitted
  diseases), 18
steps lists
  8 steps to the Low GI
    Eating Plan, 154–83
  8 steps to making a healthy
    baby, 36
  4 steps to optimizing
    pregnancy weight gain,
    69–72
  13 steps to growing a
    healthy baby, 118
stillbirths
  alcohol and risk of, 53
  exercise for prevention
    of, 16
  high-protein diets and risk
    of, 68
  listeriosis and risk of, 9,
    31, 50
  protein supplements and
    risk of, 68
  smoking and risk of, 15, 55
stock for soups, 195
stress and insulin, 111, 116
sudden infant death
  syndrome (SIDS), 15, 55,
    132, 301
summer menus, 210–11
sun exposure, 48

super foods for pregnancy, 206
  calcium super foods, 208
  folate super foods, 207
  iodine super foods, 209
  iron super foods, 207
  omega-3 fats super foods,
    208
  vitamin D super foods, 209
supplements, 32–33, 49
  and fertility, 32–33
  fish oil supplements, 44,
    127, 170
  herbal supplements, 33, 54,
    131, 179
  and pregnancy weight
    gain, 68
  prenatal vitamin and
    mineral supplements,
    32, 49
  protein supplements, 27,
    68, 76
  reviewing pre-pregnancy, 18
  See also folate or folic acid;
    iodine; iron; omega-3
    fats; entries starting with
    "vitamin"
sushi, 28, 47
symbol, GI. See GI symbol

T
tahini, 198
tea. See coffee and tea
teen pregnancy and calcium
  intake, 45
testing for gestational diabetes,
  8, 75, 99–100, 105–7
theanine, 177
"30 minutes a day rule," 93–94
this for that (replacing high
  GI with low GI foods),
    30, 77, 174–75
thyroid and thyroid
  hormones, 26
thyroxine, 46
tofu. See soy products
tomatoes, sun-dried, 196
tomato purée, 196
tongue-thrust reflex, 144
toxoplasmosis, 9, 31, 50
trans fats, 28–29, 169
tuna, canned, 194. See also
    mercury
TV viewing, 148
twins and weight gain, 72
type 1 diabetes, 8, 98, 130
type 2 diabetes, 8, 98–99
  breastfeeding as
    preventative, 125
  child's risk of due to
    mother's diet, 13, 14, 75

# Index of recipes